THE VOICE OF
NEUROSIS

THE VOICE OF
NEUROSIS

By Paul J. Moses, M.D.

*Assistant Clinical Professor in Charge of Speech and
Voice Section, Division of Otolarynology,
Stanford University School of Medicine,
San Francisco, California.*

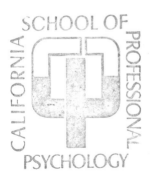

GRUNE & STRATTON   New York   1954

First printing, *June 1954*
Second printing, *June 1971*

© 1954 by Paul J. Moses, M.D.

Grune & Stratton, Inc.
757 Third Avenue, New York, New York 10017.

Library of Congress Catalog Card Number, 54-8213
International Standard Book Number, 0-8089-0334-9

Printed in the United States of America (G-B)

Contents

THE VOICE OF
NEUROSIS

Introduction

WHOEVER DIAGNOSES NEUROSIS is consciously or unconsciously affected by the patient's voice. The man who is afraid will show it in his voice as well as in his posture, gait, gestures and through what he says. Voice is the primary expression of the individual, and even through voice alone the neurotic pattern can be discovered.

In 1940 the author analyzed the voice of an adolescent from a phonograph record without having seen the individual. In doing this he developed a new category of acoustic dimensions. His description of this person compared favorably with the outcome of the Rorschach test. This was done as part of a study conducted under the auspices of the University of California Study of Adolescents (Institute of Child Welfare[1-8]). Although it was a first attempt, the following surprising correlation existed between vocal analysis and Rorschach test (*V*, voice; *R*, Rorschach):

Emotional Reactivity

V: Fearfulness, cowardice, sensitivity recognized as dominant factors. Lacking in whole-hearted enthusiasm.

R-1: Great tension arises from conflict between opposing tendencies (see below under *Direction of Emotional Adjustments*). A labile affectivity is shown, with a stabilizing factor in his strong inner life and his superior intellectual interests; through these he is able to hide his conflicts from general public view. He is irritable, however, and has great difficulty in making an effortless and satisfactory adjustment.

R-2: Inadequacy feelings. Imbalance and instability are shown in the expression of affective energy.

Direction of Emotional Adjustments

V: Autistic, schizoid, egocentric. A sadistic component is also noted, with infantile destructiveness. Self-consciousness, rigidity. Schizoid tendencies are confirmed by an epileptic-like speech melody, and a desire to avoid emotionally provocative situations.

1

R-1:   Inhibitory tendencies are in conflict with a tendency to "let go." He hesitates between an active outgoing attitude and one of submission and resignation.

R-2:   Withdrawn behavior, and also a tendency to primitive impulsive outlets. Egocentric. He shows too much fantasy to take unhealthful directions.

Social Relationships

V: Effeminate. He thinks about himself and makes himself the center of his world, playing a self-conscious social role, in expectation of a response from his audience. Histrionic, sometimes pompous. Ambitious in an unsocial way. While appearing to withdraw, he is not solitary but needs people if only to use them as objects for sadistic expression ("to show them up, tease and torment them.")

R-1:   Effeminate. Adapts to environment less by self-control than by cautious cleverness and affectation. Direct emotional relations to environment are less well organized than his "inner life."

R-2:   Social withdrawal.

Intellectual Functions

V: Intelligent and gifted, but not precise in his work. He is autistic in his thinking, with a "dance macabre" of fantastic ideas.

R-1:   Superior intelligence. He shows creative imagination and has a productive inner life. His performance, however, is uneven because of the influence of emotional tensions. Underlying conflicts affect his fundamental attitude toward the world and toward his own future.

R-2:   Above average intelligence. Shows a generalizing, abstract approach but with a capacity to see detail. Is apt to react uncritically, with a loose control over method which produces bizarre associations.

The conclusions of the vocal analysis were based upon the following classification system:

1. Level of form   good
2. Range   b flat –d
3. Symmetry   fair

4. Basic pitch	b flat
5. Key	d minor
6. Prevalent register	(pure) chest
7. Emphasis	indistinct
8. Stress	fair
9. Pathos	exaggerated
10. Speed	quiet
11. Pauses between words	smeared
12. Melody	marked
13. Uniformity-monotony	often uniform
14. Respiration	audible, irregular
15. Pitch of final syllables	going up
16. Quality	fair
17. Exactness	fair
18. Melisms	mannerisms instead
19. Loudness	normal
20. Rhythmical prevalence	yes. But "*minus* classification"
21. Melodious prevalence	no. But singsong quality evident
22. Precise speech	smeared and pasty
23. Individualities	feminisms
24. Nasal resonance	only faked
25. "Glissando"	marked

From these categories the individual was described as follows:

Analysis and Interpretation of Voice Record

This young man has a low voice with a considerable chest register. However, he does not mix his registers, but exhibits a pure chest quality and then "breaks" or switches into an almost pure head register.

Precision: There is hardly one good quality in his utterances. Lapses are shown in reading and story telling, and the pronunciation is careless except when he is self-consciously performing. The connections of words are usually "smeared," and the total impression from his speech is conveyed by such adjectives as "pasty," "dirty," and "sticky."

Insincerity and fearfulness or cowardice are revealed as dominant factors, through the absence of relation between pitch at the beginning and at the end of sentence. Effeminacy is indicated by a "glissando," avoiding concentration on one single pitch.

Self-consciousness, awareness of audience: The exaggerated duration of vowels ("Isn't that straaaaange?") reveals the expectation of reaction from the listener. It may be noted also that while some accents are over-emphasized, there is no genuine support for such emphasis; it is super-ficial and not confirmed by underlying factors. There is no vocal expres-sion of whole-hearted enthusiasm. His pathos tries to move others to sympathy, but unsuccessfully; the playing with registers is too obvious. The ending pitch of the words and sentences never fits into the melody—hence the impression of what may be called "stickiness." The content of his speech (a certain pomposity in emphasizing a psychological theme) shows a consciousness of staying in the focus of psychological observa-tion. He very cleverly takes care of satisfying both the testing recorder by a performance, and the psychologist by providing him with partly honest and partly faked material; he does not realize that his deceptions are a more reliable source of clues, although a less favorable index to his personality characteristics.

Evidences of withdrawal: The speech melody has a tendency to lower into the "lowest depths." These are like hiding places, and the whole procedure reminds one of withdrawal. There is also a sadistic component suggested by the raising and sudden lowering of the melody.

A certain rigidity, effeminate mannerisms, "not being able to stop," the course of strange ideas, and a kinship to an epileptic speech melody, indicate that we face in this record a decidedly schizoid character. Infer-ences as to most probable somatic make-up: asthenic body structure; egg-shaped face; pale complexion; long, narrow hands; moist palms; thin fingers. From the audible respiration we may infer a relatively small chest diameter. The epileptic-like speech melody suggests the possibility of temporary attacks (convulsions) in childhood.

The schizoid interpretation is also supported by the course of his thought, which is purely "autistic," in the sense in which Bleuler uses this term. He thinks about himself and makes himself the center of the world. He is boundlessly sensitive. He is, however, not solitary, for he needs people around, if only to show them up and tease or torment them. The "dance macabre" of his fantastic ideas reveals the symptoms of an infantile destructiveness.

Practical abilities: He is intelligent and gifted, but not precise in his work. He is also ambitious in an unsocial way.

This relatively crude analysis was done fifteen years ago. Since that time the author has been developing and perfecting the analysis of the personality from the voice. Currently he is doing intensive analysis of neurotic and psychotic voices as part of a research project. This project is being conducted by Gregory Bateson under a grant from the Rockefeller Foundation. Because of the close co-operation of the staff of this research project in their investigation of the paradoxes involved in communication, the author has been led to a greater understanding of the voice and its relationship to the verbal statement. He has found that one of the functions of the voice is to indicate the way verbal statements are to be interpreted. Often the vocal and verbal expression contradict each other, and when this occurs the voice is more likely to reveal the truth about the personality of the speaker.

The understanding of voice as primary expression is of importance not only to those working with vocal pathology, but to those dealing with the individual from a psychiatric point of view.

Voice analysis is of use to the psychiatrist in his diagnostic efforts. The psychoanalyst is in even greater need of an understanding of vocal features. Because of his frequent position behind the patient, the analyst depends predominantly on the expression of the patient's voice rather than on facial expression.

One might expect the laryngologist to be as interested in the emotional disturbance of laryngeal function as he is in structural pathology. Unfortunately, hardly the first steps in this direction have been taken in his training.

It is extremely difficult to draw a line between the functional and the organic. Neurotic misuse of the voice, even emotions concurrent with imaginary situations, may irritate the vocal apparatus to the point of producing organic symptoms. The opposite is also true. Organic lesions may induce psychological processes that leave scars and stimulate dysfunctions. It seems as if even the term "psychosomatic" contains too much of the old dichotomy. Psychosomatic processes do not take place in one direction only. They are not one-way streets; not even two-lane roads. They are complex mazes for which Ariadne's guiding thread has yet to be found. Usually medical evidence has to be seen or felt, and the search for facts has been primarily along visual and tactile lines. This point of view is obviously absurd when applied to disorders of the voice and yet, unfortunately, it is in existence. Notwithstanding theories, there is a certain resistance on the part of many practitioners to complaints whose causes cannot be seen or palpated.

Symptoms which are heard are just as important for the laryngologist as are symptoms which are explainable by visible factors. This principle must govern the physician concerned with voice disorders and it is from this point that his research and his therapy must begin.

Functional disorders in general are characterized by hyperfunctions or by hypofunctions of vocal muscles, or by a combination of both.[4] Without going into detail, functional disturbances may come from a variety of conditions. The energy potential of an individual may be lowered during or after some acute disease and this could make vocal expression taxing. The individual may be affected by endocrine changes which govern secondary sex organs, as in puberty, menarche, menopause. Mutational disturbances are often due to temporary strain during rearrangement of muscular coordination. Acute localized diseases can render functioning of the larynx difficult for a time and the individual can develop inefficient use of his larynx during this period and retain these habits after the acute condition disappears. And, finally, overexertion may be the result of bad training, imitation of poor examples in the environment, or lack of training where the voice is used excessively.

However, there are functional disorders which do not have such histories, or if they have, the symptoms show resistance to routine treatment. It is in such cases that the laryngologist must step into the realm of psychiatry and psychotherapy because it would be a technical impossibility to consult the psychiatrist for each of this group of patients.

The training of the psychiatrist does not contain the analysis of the voice, and the training of the laryngologist does not include sufficient psychiatric understanding of the emotional problems which affect the voice. It is hoped that this book will fill a gap related to these fields as well as to the realms of the speech and voice teacher. In addition, the crucial problems for the teacher of singing is the effect of emotional disturbances on the voice, and this book should bring him to the realization of that fact.

CHAPTER I

Fundamentals of Vocal Analysis

TODAY, POETS ARE BETTER JUDGES of the elusive products of the larynx than many of us who claim the scientific approach. The intuition of poets is keen, their responses sensitive, and they grasp the meaning of the totality, the "Gestalt," expressed by the voice. The complexity of elements that form a particular human voice, their multiplicity and individuality make analysis extremely difficult.

Science has not yet developed a fully acceptable method of voice analysis. This is not astonishing; other branches of personality research are in their infancy too. Physiology has wide, unexplored gaps, and we are just beginning to scratch the surface in the complicated field of psychosomatics.

Since Quintilian,[5] who was the first to describe vocal function according to quantity and quality of voices (first century A. D.), philosophers, phoneticians, and physicians have puzzled over the problem of the human voice. Little has been accomplished, however, in the study of the voice as a key to personality: normal, neurotic or psychotic. The derivation of the word "personality" proves that there was originally a profound understanding of the close connection between voice and personality. The word comes from the Latin *persona,* which originally meant the mouthpiece of a mask used by actors (*per sona:* the sound of the voice passes through). From the mask the term shifted to the actor; the "person" in a drama. The word eventually came to mean any person and finally "personality," but over the centuries it lost its symbolic connection with the voice.

This book will reverse the history of the word "persona." Again the voice will stand for the person whom it expresses. We are surrounded by the mouthpieces of masks in all the modern devices of communication: radio, telephone, movies, television. To learn what is behind the mask, we have to learn to use more than intuition.

How intuition operates can be illustrated by a rather trivial ex-

7

ample. Every experienced physician who receives an "urgent" night call knows how soon he should see his patient simply by his reaction to the voice, not the words. This instinctive reaction is an undifferentiated impression, the result of former experiences. It is a complex psychological process made up of everything that happens to us when we hear a voice for the first time, or, as in this example, a voice under justified or neurotic anxiety.

Intuitive judgment depends largely on association. This includes emotional reaction to voices one likes or dislikes. The voice of one person reminds us of someone else, and this calls up visual images and other sense impressions with agreeable or disagreeable associations. Many persons compare the voices they hear with their own, without knowing that they do so. "It is too loud for me" often means "It is too loud in comparison with my own voice."

Medical analysis of voice requires more precise tools than intuitive response. Something objective, something which can be verified by others, must be found.

Before attempting to analyze voice, one must divorce it from the message it seeks to convey and release it as far as is possible from the bondage of subjective association. In this day of radio and television we are exposed to a constant torrent of voices. To listen to a news broadcast we have learned unconsciously to extinguish the voice and concentrate on what it transmits. In scientific vocal analysis we must reverse the procedure: subtract the content and retain the voice impression.

The next step is to describe a voice as objectively as possible, avoiding subjective value judgments of bad or good. The first difficulty arises here because nomenclature is virtually nonexistent for expressing the primary perception of vocal phenomena. Other fields of sense impression are less handicapped. Terms for colors are generally accepted and a painting, therefore, can be described in terms which convey color impressions and nothing else. But to describe a voice, words must be borrowed from the experience of other sense organs. We speak of a black basso, light baritone, or a high soprano. This borrowing is "synaesthesia," a mixture of sensory impressions belonging to different sense departments. The best known is "colored hearing." However, this terminology, although generally accepted, is useless for objective analysis.

Another handicap of nomenclature is the lack of common language used in different approaches: singing teachers of various schools used different terms, terms which are not used by laryngologists, who in turn differ from speech teachers, phoneticians and music critics. It is this discrepancy of language which has hampered the cooperation of the professions in spite of common interests.

Since the laryngologist's approach is predominantly visual, he often describes laryngeal function from a more mechanical point of view. He depends on the larynx mirror which reveals closing and opening functions of vocal cords, their color, and possible thickening and tumors. Consistency of tissue, humidity or dryness, dislocation in vertical direction, coordination between internal and external muscle fibers remain unnoticed. The terms "hoarse" or "husky" have become standard description of dysfunctions.

The terminology lacks standards, but the phenomena are so complex that they defy simple designations. Terms such as warm, cold, hard, soft, sharp, wooden, metallic have no place in an objective description of the voice. They show how little progress has been made in auditory observation.

Contemporary research approaches voice analysis in three different ways: through the listener's perception, through visual observation, and through acoustic examination. The first type of research is mainly concerned with what the voice itself is and with how the hearer experiences the voice. Pear[6] in England and Bühler[7] in Austria conducted large-scale studies over the radio in which listeners guessed the age, weight, sex and occupation of the person whose voice they heard. Cantril and Allport[8] in the United States approached the problem somewhat differently, giving more scope to free expression of the listener's judgment. They used the matching technique. Judges who heard the voice of a speaker stated their impressions of his physical and psychological traits. These experiments were on the basis of impression: which voice belonged with which traits? No objective analysis of voice was applied, and associations with former experiences were used exclusively. Many psychology departments in colleges have continued investigations along these lines. Sanford[9] states that agreement among judges was often greater than their accuracy. He blames this on stereotyped standards. The relative worthlessness of these studies shows that intuition is based on experience, that piping little voices were associated with children, baritone voices with men, hesitation in speech with shyness. They also reveal a socio-cultural bias dominating our interpretations.

Whatever the psychological or sociological value of these listening studies may be, they do not furnish us with the much-needed tools of vocal analysis. Their supposition is the same as ours: namely, that vocal dynamics mirror psychodynamics. However, the problem cannot be approached on the level of impressions and trying to sense through intuition the specific voice of a specific personality.

Visual methods of observation have been used for many years in vocal analysis.[10] We seem to grasp the component meanings of complex entities and their interrelations easier when we can see them on a graph. Air movement measurements during respiration and phonation, oscillations of tones, and speech melodies and rhythms can be shown precisely in graphs. The visual method has contributed greatly to vocal analysis by separating the voice from content and by establishing objective, measurable units of observation. In this way analytical procedure escapes undifferentiated subjective intuition and the pitfalls of socially predetermined bias.

While the visual method successfully isolates certain elements of the voice, it cannot be applied to other elements. Its greatest weakness is that the parts remain apart and do not integrate themselves into a comprehensive picture of the whole. This severely limits the areas of interpretation. The connection between personality and its expression becomes lost in the maze of detail.

Acoustic examination plays a strange part in medicine. Medical students learn to listen to the sounds of heart and lungs. But they are not supposed to trust their ears without the help of visual criteria, such as x-rays and electrocardiograms. The same thing occurs in experimental phonetics, where the main characteristics of speech and voice details are established by ear, but where one feels safe only by transferring these details to graphs.

One objection to a broader application of acoustic examination is that listening is both subjective and unreliable. The answer is that in this type of investigation the ears of the examiner must be trained to perceive, to remember, to interpret. Acoustic methods are blamed for revealing totality instead of parts. But through training we can learn to listen to many constituent voice elements, such as pitch, intensity, and duration. For more exact analysis these elements do need to be transformed into graphic presentations.

Grasping the whole of a phenomenon is essential in the scientific approach.[11] The whole is a firm anchor to reality. Parts have no life and no meaning without it. The parts must be isolated for the sake of analysis, but we should always remember that this is an artificial process. Without a thorough understanding of the relation of parts to the whole, which entails an understanding of the whole as well, no synthesis and no creation is possible.

Acoustic examination must take its legitimate place among scientific processes, but it needs great development before it can rank with visual methods. To perceive the human voice correctly and to conceive the right inferences, the listener must acquire, must train himself in, "creative hearing."

Let us use a simple example to explain creative hearing. In a concert the tenor delivers an aria in a throaty voice. After a short time the audience becomes restless. One person after another begins to clear his throat and one would think there was a cold epidemic. This is what actually happened: The tenor narrowed his throat. His tongue went backward to his pharyngeal wall—and simply through listening many individuals were affected. Their tongues went back slightly, creating a certain dryness, and this caused them to clear their throats. In "creative hearing" the reflex muscular reaction of listening must be brought into consciousness. The spontaneous and sympathetic kinesthetic sensation which occurs in the muscular functions of the listener's apparatus must be recognized.

The best explanation of the phenomenon "creative hearing" comes from Bernfeld's theories on "fascination"[12]: Primitive perception is close to motor reaction. The primitive ego imitates that which is perceived in an attempt to master intense stimuli. "Perceiving and changing one's own body according to what is perceived were originally one and the same thing."

Creative hearing stems from the roots of fascination, but it is raised to the level of consciousness. It is an audiokinetic method of examination. While it is an unfamiliar approach, it should not be impulsively rejected. Bringing motor reactions into consciousness is not much different from, and no less reliable than, becoming conscious of visual or auditive reactions.

For understanding the voice of the neurotic and psychotic person, creative hearing is of paramount importance. In the neurotic individual, pantomimic movements are more pronounced than under normal conditions. This is also true of the congenitally deaf individual who, unless he is educated, does not think in words but rather in terms of events or states as a whole. To analyze events into their component parts and then give a separate symbol of hand and mouth to each component is a comparatively new development in the life of the human species. Cries of pleasure and distress probably preceded pantomimic speech, while vocalizing in imitation of natural phenomena must have been simultaneous with the development of speech. Paget[13] explains how mouth gestures in speech—our articulation—were originally associated with pantomime gestures. The changes of our laryngeal organs are now associated with changes in our facial expression. If this theory of the origin of language is sound, then creative hearing merely reverses the process by analyzing gestures that create sound: that is, it "reads" the sounds, not by ear but kinesthetically. The correlation between these pantomimic expressions is important in interpreting regression to primordial or infantile patterns in psychopathological conditions.

It should be re-emphasized that creative hearing is not the same as intuition. Intuition is, and by definition remains, undifferentiated. It is unconscious and subjective; i.e., not verifiable by others. Creative hearing is conscious; it may be used as an analytical tool to observe elements of voice singly and in relation to each other and to the whole; and furthermore, it can be verified. We have today kymographs and other devices to record voices, and the records can be examined at will. Observations can be repeated as often as necessary and by as many analysts as may wish to do so. Some voice elements can be translated into visual records for further checking if this seems desirable.

According to Bühler,[14] who conducted some of the first audience studies, a human utterance whether it be speaking, singing, or a simple ejaculation, has three functions:

1. Representation. It tells something.
2. Expression. It reveals something about the speaker.
3. Appeal. It wants to—and does—elicit a reaction from the listener.

When a man on the streetcar suddenly addresses his neighbor with the remark, "Awful weather!", he does not intend representing a fact which was unknown before. He is appealing for a reaction on the part of any listener to avoid loneliness.

In voice analysis, we must divorce ourselves from the first function, which relates to content. The main body of observation must be directed toward the second function, that of expression. Appeal should be considered in areas of interpretation where it is pertinent; for instance, under psychotic conditions with their varieties of communication behavior, appeal can be the center of vocal investigation. The schizophrenic voice often has a typical monologue character— as if the partner in a conversation is not addressed at all. This phenomenon is caused by absence of appeal dimensions.

What does the voice reveal about the speaker? How does voice convey that totality which is the neurotic individual? To what conditions and processes in his physiology and psychology does voice relate?[15]

The word "analysis" has been used very loosely in studies relating to voice. For example, in the "personality description" studies, even when conducted by such an outstanding psychologist as Werner Wolff,[16, 17] the listener does not analyze the voice he hears or the personality of the speaker. He analyzes his own reactions to the voice. One wonders whether it is appropriate to apply the word "analysis" to the listing of a limited number of free associations or to guessing answers to a few specified questions.

Analysis means resolving an entity into its constituent elements so that they reveal their relations to one another and to the whole. For this we must first find a way to isolate the elements of the voice. Priority will be given here to those factors which we suspect have significant correlation with other important functions of the body and mind of the neurotic. Second, we must describe these elements in measurements or other unambiguous, verifiable terms. Third, we should trace the influences that shape any observed variations. And finally, we should be able to integrate these parts into meaningful patterns.

Certain vocal features stand out in bold relief while others assume significance only in relationships. Some are primary physiological functions and others are products of complex cortical organization.

CHAPTER II

Vocal Ontogenesis,
The Blueprint for Neurotic Patterns

VOICE IS AN INDICATOR of different phases in a person's life. It is free from static qualities. Vocal changes accompany the development of the individual, but in addition, voice contains archaic properties originating in the cradle of mankind. One can go so far as to say that vocal expression is a record of the history of mankind as well as a record of the individual. It contains phylogenetic and ontogenetic material. Modern psychopathology has taught us that neurotic patterns are characterized by fixation and regression, with the implication that the individual is fixed to a certain phase in his own development or goes back to a previous, mostly infantile phase of his own life. The basic difference between the neurotic and the schizophrenic patient is audible in vocal expression: the neurotic voice reveals typical symptoms of fixation and regression through vocal patterns belonging to earlier phases in his development, whereas the schizophrenic voice has a marked archaic character, with primordial attributes (see Conclusion).

It is therefore necessary for the understanding of the neurotic voice to be familiar with the ontogenetic development of voice in general. Thinkers of the past have been much intrigued by the fact that the first manifestation of human life is vocal. The chronicles of sixteenth-century Spanish monks record an ancient interpretation: The first cry of the child expresses sorrow and reproach. The new-born boy cries, "O-Ah," and the girl "O-Eh," abbreviating the Latin words "O Adam (O Eve), *cur peccavisti?*"; "O Adam, (O Eve) Why did you sin?" The belief that a child's sex can be determined from his first cry has been and is still part of the folklore of many ethnic groups.

Immanuel Kant devoted a whole chapter of his *Anthropologie,*

15

written in 1789, to the first cry of the infant. In his opinion the child feels the fetters nature imposed on him; he rebels against his inability to control his body and cries out in anguish and resentment. Kant believed that humans were the only species which emitted a sound at birth and thought this an extremely dangerous trait, as in a wild state of life it might reveal the hiding place of the mother, weakened by labor, and make her and the newborn an easy prey to hunting carnivores. Kant therefore supposed that the birth cry developed in a period when humanity had reached a degree of social organization adequate to protect the mother and the newborn. Debates on the infant's cry went on, however. Michelet, Hegel's pupil, interpreted the first cry as the reflection of the "horror of the spirit at its subjection to nature."

The physiological facts are less romantic. The glottis is obstructed by mucus and opens forcefully. By the audible cry the respiratory tract is cleared for the first breath. It is also a reflex to the brutal shock of temperature change, of light, and fresh air. No gene structures controlling the larynx development of the sexes have been found. All infants, male or female, emit similar sounds: a monotonous wail around the pitch of a'-b'. The intuitive impression has always interpreted these cries as expression of displeasure and discomfort, therefore close to protest, an important pattern formation.

Early in the baby's existence—between the second and fourth week—the mother can tell from his cry whether he is hungry, wet, or just bored.[18] Not that the baby intentionally communicates his needs. In this "crying period" he emits about six to eight half tones in the middle soprano range. These sounds, repeated over and over again have some rhythmic and melodious features and are interspersed with high notes, occasionally as high as "c." The infant makes these sounds in reflex to various stimuli—as genuine a self-expression, as true a monologue, as one ever encounters. He expresses moods, needs, reactions, without yet aiming at or asking for anything. He cries softly when not uncomfortable and employs a harder attack when displeased. Lamentation is characterized by a falling pitch.

In crying, the pattern of fast inspiration and long, slow expiration becomes set, and later this becomes the prototype of the breathing function employed in speaking. The difference between pleasurable and displeasurable respiration becomes noticeable in infants.

The infant probably reproduces in his development the path that humanity as a species traveled. His vocal powers first develop a marked degree of expressiveness. Then, as articulation takes over, the function of the voice becomes less dominant and more subtly complex.

The newborn enters an empty world. Nothing reminds him of previous experience, except perhaps rhythm, to which he became conditioned through his mother's pulse beat and mother's respiration in his intrauterine life. He has no memories which could help him to differentiate sounds or to visualize events connected with sounds. On the contrary, the source of all future acoustic associations is the slowly developing identification of mother's voice with food, warmth, comfort—a musical background to pleasure sensations.

The child is also born with certain inclinations and capacities. Actions and traits which do not have to be taught to him are termed "genotypical," while the expressions he has to learn from others, especially his mother, are called "phenotypical." Playing with lips, with vocal cords, with the tongue are genotypical actions. The first laughter of the baby is also considered a self-taught manifestation. It goes without saying that the establishment of phenotypical functions is an indicator of the attention and protection which the child receives from his mother. Anxiety neurosis of the child, which can be the result of an unsatisfied need for protection, will be expressed through vocal patterns which originate at this time. It will reveal itself by insufficient coordination between respiration and phonation.

Sometime during the second and third month of life the baby discovers that the sounds he himself makes have the power to conjure up mother's presence. At the magic command of this unique tool, food, dry diapers, sucking pleasure, soothing sounds, rocking and other delights materialize. He finds that he can "influence people," attract them or shy them away by the use of his voice. From then on the infant's cry is purposeful, and as such, a certain kind of speech.

The three fundamental emotions of fear, rage and love have even

at this early stage of life specific vocal expressions. Fear is indicated
by a sudden catching of breath, a puckering of lips, and a certain
quality of crying; rage by screaming and breathholding until the face
is crimson. Love, if one may call such the reactions to the stroking
of the erogenous zones and to gentle rocking and soothing sounds,
is expressed by soft sounds, cooing and gurgling. It is interesting
to observe the body movements coincidental with these sounds: in
fear shrinking and an attempt to decrease the body surface; in rage,
spasticity; and when expressing love, relaxed reaching movements,
the forerunners of embracing, or at least a widening manifestation.

The organs of speech, from vocal cords to lips, have a discharging
function, and the movements of these organs are therefore libidinal
in character. In other words, the production of sounds and noises
takes place in conjunction with pleasing body sensations. Eating and
chewing are accompanied by grunts and smacks, and these sounds
become impregnated with pleasure sensations.

It is during this early period that the "body language" of allergy
first manifests itself. For example, the baby might express protest
against being deprived of mother's milk by the only means he has,
his body, and rashes will appear on his skin after the first mouthful
of cereal or egg. Breathholding is as much of a somatic expression
of emotion as is constipation. Stridor of the larynx is a rather frightening spastic condition which often glides into symptoms of pseudo-
croup or, in later years, of asthma. Just the same, it is an expression
of frustration and protest. If this kind of vocal "trick" provokes
a special alarm reaction from the parents, it may develop, completely
unconsciously, into an automatic habit pattern designed to gain
attention.

Around the fourteenth week the infant begins to produce sounds
that resemble singing. What has started as a reflex now becomes a
play pattern. He vocalizes, he laughs loudly. The range of his voice
expands and the dynamics become more pronounced. When he is
about six months old, the baby enters the second stage of vocal
development, the lalling period. He is just learning to control his
arms and legs at will, and now he begins to experiment with his
mouth and tongue. He moves his lips and his tongue rhythmically

and starts lalling: "da-da-da," "la-la-la." He does not want to communicate, he does not yet imitate sounds he hears; he just wants the pleasure sensation of repeating simple syllables and rhythmically touching smaller or wider areas of mucous membranes. This is an outer erotization coupled with motor and acoustic sensations, a triple enjoyment. Repeating syllables is a basic primitive sound formation. It is easier than rearranging the muscles in a new coordination to obtain new consonants, and the rhythm of repetition helps to engrave the sound as well as the motor pattern on the child's brain centers. At this point the distinctly rhythmic features of the schizophrenic in motor pattern and especially in speech behavior should be mentioned.

Children all over the world, irrespective of their parents' language, develop articulation in the same sequence: from lips (P, B, M) to the tip of the tongue (T, D, L, N) to the back of the tongue (K, G). Lalling is the dress-rehearsal for later articulation; a rhythmic conditioning of the motor center for subsequent volitional production of imitative sounds. But lalling has other functions too. Singing satisfies a narcissistic libido. Lalling is an oral satisfaction of a higher level than sucking. It is almost an artistic phenomenon. The child feels, produces, hears, and repeats. He enjoys oral movement, rhythm and sound.

Perhaps it is because voice production in this wordless age leaves solely agreeable memories that we have the urge later in life to sing when we are happy and gay.

Voice production in this vocal age is practically unlimited. Happiness and displeasure can be expressed over endless periods; no hoarseness will interfere. The breathing capacity does not seem to have limits; it functions ideally—a trait which, unfortunately, will soon be lost. If the same child takes singing lessons eighteen years later, it will be only with great difficulty that some of this ideal breathing and phonation is regained. This is because speech and articulation have been superimposed and interfere with free functioning of the vocal cords and with free breathing. Voice becomes subordinated to speech until it is merely an emotional background which we disregard as we do music in the movies. The better the movie's musical score, the less attention we pay to it. We notice it only when it does not fit the words and the action on the screen. This same discrepancy one finds in schizophrenics who might accompany the gay content of a story with a sad voice and the tragic content with a merry one.

During the lalling period the child begins to recognize mother's voice. It emerges distinctly from the musical background to pleasure and comfort. Because of the simultaneous development of hearing and voice, it is especially important that mothers encourage babies in lalling. Mothers also prompt the child's transition into the next vocal stage by singing to them. Infants are sensitive to music. It is not unusual for them to sing before they speak. They will repeat whole musical phrases heard from their mothers—or from radio commercials.

"Echolalia" means repetition of sounds, syllables and words that are not understood. How long an infant will continue doing so will depend on his speech impulses and his ability to understand what is said to him. Children with low speech impulse or an early understanding of words will indulge less in echolalia. It is physiologically a means of developing tone and word memory as well as word understanding and that is why environmental influences help set a child's vocal pattern in this early, imitative period. No doubt the interpersonal family relation with and around the child plays a significant part. Echolalia becomes a pathological, almost pathognomic symptom in schizophrenia. Lacking object relation, the patient cannot disconnect himself from a word. He may repeat a question again and again or repeat a word in the same meaningless way with the same intonation over and over.

The baby lives in a world of his own before he is able to think verbally. He "thinks" through emotions. He does not possess words but has a voice to express emotions. Although it is considered remote from logic, Fenichel, nevertheless, calls it thinking because it consists of imagination and is the same basic process by which later actions are performed. It is carried out through pictorial images and resembles primitive magical thought. Similarities are not distinguished from identities; the object and the picture are equated. By self-identification, what happens to the contemplated object is experienced as if it were happening to the Ego. Ego and Non-Ego are not yet separated. The child still has not grasped that there is a reality outside itself. Again the correlation of normal development with later schizophrenic thinking is brought to mind. It is not surprising that schizophrenic thinking, which has regressed to this infantile level, will be expressed by vocal means whose pattern was similarly set in childhood.

From this maze of self-identification the child slowly emerges to the realization of distinct entities around him. Because his thinking is emotional, he grasps the emotions that surround him and he does this through the voices he hears. Just as a dog obeys his master without understanding the articulatory part of the words but catches the melody and the dynamic accents, the child in this wordless period senses the moods of his parents and reacts to soothing words and to irritating approaches. This gives us the key to the neurotic reaction to situations which the child could not possibly "understand" logically, as for instance, the imminent separation of his parents or worry about a sick member of the family.

Chapter III will describe how reaction to rhythm is established in children before melody leaves any impression on them at all. Acoustic perception in an infant has motor associations. He will, therefore, try to transform acoustic experiences into motor experiences. This was described in Chapter I as "fascination." The urge and "talent" for dancing in feeble-minded children up to about ten years of age is due to this cause.

In this complicated period of wordless give and take many later traits become established for better or for worse. Superimposed on the baby's uninhibited, original vocal manifestations are the acoustic impressions identified with the moods of others, and the kinetic compulsion of fascination to recreate the sounds heard. The result is that the child, and later the adult, is impressed as he expresses. In other words, he will emit a certain sound when frightened, and from then on, whenever he hears this sound it will mean "fright" to him. Any other way of expressing fright will be foreign. This particularly explains our reactions to voices later in life. For example, in certain cultures, raising of the voice is natural and does not imply anger or command. But the Anglo-American outlook may make us misinterpret the spirited disputation of, for instance, a Spaniard, as being agitation, emotional imbalance, or even a temper tantrum! Linguistics records parallel experience. Provincial people mistrust "foreigners" who speak in a different dialect or with a different accent from the one prevailing in the immediate neighborhood. Patterns differing from one's own are accepted only after being exposed to experiences that effectively widen the horizons of vocal understanding. This mistrust often degenerates into paranoid behavior.

An essential part of infantile and archaic thinking is experiencing the world in symbols. This primitive symbolism is part of prelogical thinking and is not to be confused with the symbolic distortions of neurotics and psychotics. It is not strictly in accordance with reality but is governed by wishful imagining. It is preparation for the real control of environment. The child retraces ontogenetically in his own development the road that humanity traveled from magic to the real mastery of reality. To be able to establish this, to differentiate successfully between the individual and his environment, between reality and imagination, between the conscious and the unconscious, he needs the decisive tools: words. The faculty of speech changes pre-thought into a logical, organized process adjusted to reality.

The child first speaks one-word sentences and then he makes the transition to more complex expressions. He does not describe things with his first words but makes his wishes and feelings known. These early stages of speech are impregnated with musical-vocal elements because the indications of wishes and feelings demand dynamic and melodious accents. The child at this time learns the different functions of quiet respiration, through the nose with small amounts of air, and speech respiration, deep voluntary inspiration through the mouth, using a greater volume of air. It is intriguing to note how soon a small child learns to gauge the exact amount of air he needs. It is just as interesting to observe how quickly the neurotic will leave this well-learned pattern and eventually be unable to anticipate the volume of air he needs to finish a sentence.

Some speech difficulties may start at this period. The child wishes to express something for which his vocabulary is insufficient, and he stutters. Fortunately this type of stuttering (misnamed "physiological stuttering") is usually transient.[19, 20] Lisping at this age is a simple continuation of infantile oral gratification. Playing with saliva, touching mucous membranes with the tongue are among the earliest sources of pleasure. Children like to lisp because it involves a similar kind of enjoyment. Lisping may, however, be continued longer than usual, not from obstinacy, but because of a certain confusion. "Th" is a lisped "S"; and it is rather hard for the child to understand why lisping is sometimes allowed and sometimes not. It may be noted here that lisping in adults is usually fixation to this early speech level as an expression of neurotic traits.

At about eighteen months the child enters actively into the life of the family. Before this he was completely self-centered, but now he begins to recognize his mother as a person, apart from himself, and not merely as a source of food, warmth and comfort. Father and other members of the family enter the picture in a new light. But the child is still egocentric. "They" exist for him alone. Every disturbance in this anticipated self-centered relationship may result in conflict.

Children have a fine ear for insincerity in the voice, regardless of what the voice says. The so-called intuition of the small child is based on acute attention to sounds and on an equally acute interpretation of the moods that produce it. To a child, therefore, baby talk coming from the mouth of a tall adult often seems ridiculous and perhaps frightening. The false paternal inflections of the department store Santa Claus or the self-conscious physician are equally bewildering. Unconscious rejection on the part of one or both parents is divined from the voice more than from the content, and thus creates conflict even though the situation is thought by the adults to be "under control."

Many vocal disturbances have their origin in the next period of the child's life, when contemporaries, to whom he may compare himself, enter his orbit. It often takes newcomers in nursery schools several weeks to adjust before they can follow the songs, dances and recitations of the group, or before they even understand the jargon of the "initiated." This is not merely shyness but is due to the discrepancy which is experienced for the first time between the child's own individual pattern of rhythm, voice and speech and that of the group representing the outside world—not the world of adults but that of equals. Some children cannot adapt. They reject the new pattern and face conflicts, while the majority adjust gradually. In the process of adjustment, however, they often become fractious, restive, negative, a stage greatly resembling adolescence.

If we understand that this is a difficult period in the child's life, characterized by irritability and aggressiveness, it becomes clear how certain vocal symptoms develop. Spasms, disturbances in the rhythmic flow of physiological processes are probably the most general signs of somatic protests. Breath-holding and stridor of the larynx were mentioned before as spastic symptoms of rage. The noisy explosive opening of the glottis relieves aggressiveness. The child almost spits the sounds into the listener's face. Stuttering, both the tonic and clonic kind, is spastic in nature and is a neurotic reaction to circumstances to which the child objects. He knows no other way to express his objection. In this phase the child may also express his protest at having been thrust into a cold world by reverting to infantile articulatory patterns, or more simply, by refusing to speak at all.

A small child does not know of the existence of words. He thinks first in pictures and through emotions and by connecting ideas to sound sequences—sentences. Grade school opens a new portal: that of words. In the first grade the child sees for the first time words as such on the blackboard. He learns that there is a space between words, black on the board and white in the book. That formidable space between familar sounds which transforms them suddenly into words to be memorized may become a stumbling block.

Speech development and the small child's speech problems have been studied much more thoroughly than the voices of children. We know that the small child's speaking voice ranges from a' to f' sharp. His singing voice has a range of five half notes in the first and second year; ten to thirty-one by his seventh year; and by the time he reaches fifteen, his range extends from sixteen to forty-one half notes. Retarded children usually have smaller ranges than normal children. Boys' ranges are narrower than those of girls (figure 1).

Voice differences between small boys and girls have not been studied thoroughly, although it is generally believed that differences

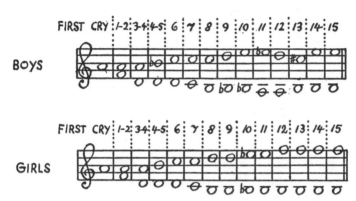

FIG. 1.—From the first cry to adolescence. Singing range of children.

begin to shape up rather early in life. Boys' voices express more aggressiveness; girls' voices show greater modulation. Mother's voice is the first mold that helps to form the child's voice, but as soon as a boy child knows his sex, he begins to copy other patterns. Little girls with dolls will display marked maternal influences in their voices, although their vocabulary may be quite inadequate and inappropriate. Little boys, on the other hand, will imitate their fathers, or preferably a radio cowboy or other such hero. Small children establish associations with radio voices early and accurately. They recognize the sheriff, the judge, the gangster, the good and the bad cowboy long before they completely or even partially understand the content of the program. In their games, children will portray these characters, not through dialogue, but by sound. They learn to imitate background noises such as airplanes, machine guns, rocket ships with frightening accuracy.

When the child enters school, his vocabulary expands and so does his range of yells, screams and other noises. However, of even greater importance, he now comes face to face with one of the greatest influences of his life: the teacher. The teacher is not only a mother substitute. She is the model. She directs, she teaches, she gives examples. She writes the school copy on the blackboard and gives the best marks to the one who makes the best copy. No wonder her voice, as well as her handwriting, is imitated. Nowadays candidates for teaching positions have to pass a speech clearance test. Those with defective speech and voice are screened out, but it is not the obvious defects that have the most detrimental effect on the pupils. Mannerisms of speech, artificiality of tone, and the cumulative frustration scarring the voice of so many women in this thankless profession are the qualities that are mirrored by the child.

That elementary school teaching is almost exclusively a female profession is recognized as a problem by experts in many different fields. It should be acknowledged that the frequency of feminine voices among American men will not be reduced and the ratio of male homosexuality will not be less as long as a boy's first real life contact with a father image is the Army Sergeant in the ROTC. Even under the best circumstances, when the family is sound and the father gives the child adequate attention, the child is still searching for "doubles" in the outside world. He finds his equals in his playmates, his mother's extension in the teacher. But there is no second to his father in the new real life environment.

There is a certain stage when the little boy will shun girl playmates in school and will seek feverishly for a masculine pattern outside the school. This is the time when sports may have an important effect on his general deportment as well as on his vocal development. Boys who belong to sandlot baseball teams or to small fry scout troops acquire with the slang of the particular group a certain manliness in their tone. They learn to catch a ball with a professional yell. The piano quality of their voices changes to fortissimo. Unfortunately, vocal virility remains too often merely a matter of increased volume. Feminine influence still prevails. The majority of males, even those in the sports groups, who come into his life at this stage do not help the boy to shape his vocal behavior into a truly masculine pattern.

The small child learns to write by imitating, but after a year or two his individuality breaks through the standardized form. The same is true of voice. With the acquisition of a vocabulary the child learns to word his experiences and these take deep memory roots. The words are accompanied by speech melody, which reflects the emotions attending the experiences, and these too are stored away. But speech melody has been stamped on the memory from earlier experiences. Family and group relationships have been symbolized by vocal patterns before verbal thinking was mastered. Love, security, frustration, anxiety have acquired their particular themes. Identification with parents or with parent substitutes molds the voice further, as do personal urges, interests and drives. The voice of the child is like a complicated engraving etched by experience with multitudinous fine traces which cannot be easily eradicated.

MUTATION

Puberty is one of the most crucial and upsetting periods in human life. It is therefore natural that the voice, which is a sensitive instrument reflecting all our experiences, physical, emotional, environmental, should register the upheaval. Puberty is not a simple change that happens overnight. It is a lengthy process, taking several years. The first phase is pubescence, when signs of disorganization are most conspicuous. The second phase is pubertal development. Then the transformation has been largely accomplished and functioning is continued on a newly organized level. Some changes still occur during this last phase, but they are more gradual, less swift. The over-all picture of the vocal apparatus at this stage shows a considerable growth and distinct reshaping. As a result the child's breathing becomes more capacious, the range of his tone wider, the resonance and power of his voice more pronounced. In most instances his speaking voice becomes deeper. This process of general voice change during puberty is termed "mutation." According to Weiss, organic and functional mutation should be considered as two theoretically independent concepts.

Slight pre-mutational voice changes may begin as early as nine years of age in girls and ten years in boys. The duration of the mutational period of the speaking voice is estimated between overnight and one year. The singing voice changes much more slowly and it may take as long as eight years before it settles to its new level.

Geography, culture and race can influence the advent and duration of mutation. Children of city dwellers and of educated parents seem to mature and mutate earlier than others.

It is necessary to throw light on different developmental features of mutation in order to understand the neurotic voice.[21, 22] Mutation marks the end of the infantile phase in vocal development and the beginning of adulthood expressed through voice. Unless one understands the physiology and pathology of mutation, it is impossible to determine the different steps of vocal regression. Of greatest importance is the so-called persistent falsetto voice, which signifies fixation of the male voice at a certain level before these physiological changes take place.

No difference has been found in the gene structures controlling the female and male larynx development. Boys and girls have a similar vocal apparatus before mutation. Puberty brings considerable changes, not only in the relative size of the vocal cords, but also in their direction of growth. The boy's larynx grows about one centimeter in an *anterior-posterior* direction, forming the Adam's apple. Girls' vocal cords grow three to four millimeters. The speaking voice of boys may drop a full octave, while that of girls may drop only a third of an octave.

Puberty affects the voice of both sexes with considerable impact because the larynx is a secondary sex organ, and all sexual development, as well as degeneration, is accompanied by modifications in the voice.[23] However, as far back as Aristotle, interest has always centered on male mutation. The reason for this is that the change in boys' voices is usually much more dramatic than the change in girls' voices. Some boys are afflicted with a sudden break in their voice, a sudden involuntary change in pitch and quality. While this is not a pathological symptom, it is by no means as common as is generally believed. In most instances mutation, both in boys and in girls, takes place gradually. It starts with a certain huskiness and the speaking voice may become unsteady. Most often the vaccilation is not more than one or two tones. This unreliability of voice production is due to the child's difficulty in coordinating the rapidly growing organs at their new level of functioning. It may happen that the voice will drop somewhat lower at first than the ultimate level at which it will stabilize. During this period the vocal cords do not close completely but form what is called the mutational triangle.

Puberty and mutation are subject to a great many other influences, among which cultural factors are not the least. In our present day Western civilization, the period of puberty is artificially prolonged because our culture makes the social and psychological adaptation to the physiological changes rather difficult and drawn out.

During periods of major endocrinological changes the individual becomes introspective. He seems compelled to concentrate on himself. He shows interest in abstractions, such as life, death, love. He wants to find himself and the meaning for his existence. Such behavior attends menopause as well as adolescence. Some authorities have also observed it during the turbulent developmental period of children in the 4 to 5 year group. In adolescence, new urges disturb the consciousness of the individual. He is full of contradictions. Sometimes he covers his deep uncertainties and anxieties with excessive rudeness and aggression.

The adolescent boy swings like a pendulum between his infantile desire for security and comfort, symbolized by his mother, and his new longing for a girl, a non-incestuous object for his sex urge. Society discourages the satisfaction of this new urge by using his female relatives as a club over his head: "Think of girls as if they were your mother or your sister." He feels guilty and is strengthened in his inclination to go back to mother. This ambivalence is expressed in his vocal behavior. He teeters precariously on the brink of heterosexuality, not knowing where to fall. Backward is mother (and homosexuality) and the clinging to a high, childish voice; forward is manhood (and The Girl) and the acceptance of his new deep voice.

Little attention and almost no research has been given over to these adjustment problems of adolescent girls, as their voice change is less audible.

But male or female, dramatic or gradual, prolonged or instantaneous, the period of puberty and mutation comes to an end. Final vocal decisions must be made in accordance with reality. When extreme ambivalence persists in a voice, it has persisted in the personality of the individual and it becomes a pathological problem. When an adult clings to a child's voice, he is endocrinologically stigmatized. Mutational pathology, including such problems as prolonged mutation and persistent falsetto voice will be discussed later, but it should be emphasized here that the overwhelming majority of mutational disturbances are due not to organic pathology but to the chaotic handling of the adolescent and his voice. An ounce of prevention would eliminate many vocal complications and subsequently the emotional conflicts which are vocally expressed.

CHAPTER III

Acoustic Dimensions of Voice: The Five R's

ACOUSTIC DIMENSIONS ARE, for the most part, measurable. They are different in nature, in significance and in effect. The one characteristic they have in common is that the trained listener can clearly identify and isolate them and that the observations of all trained listeners will coincide within close margins of error.

By coincidence the English words designating five of these acoustic dimensions start with an "R." This chance fact helped to subdivide the somewhat confusing material pertaining to the measurable features of voice.

In this chapter and the next the following attributes of voice will be described:

Acoustic Dimensions (The "Five R's")	Other Dimensions	Other Significant Features
Respiration	Melody	Pathos
Range	Intensity	Mannerism
Registers	Speed	Melism
Resonance	Accents	Exactness
Rhythm	Emphasis	Pauses between words

RESPIRATION

Sounds are produced by currents, jets, puffs, explosions and stoppages of breath. Without normal breathing there is no normal phonation. In the voice of neurosis a vocal abnormality is always accompanied by respiratory irregularities. When an adult speaks, respiration starts automatically with the intention to speak. Respiration cannot be accomplished at will without the intent to speak. The small child has to learn to anticipate the volume of breath he needs for what he wants to say, and his learning process is discernible. When this skill is not mastered so that breathing is as automatic as walking, speech difficulties result. In neurosis, when the aim of communication is ambivalent, this co-ordination will suffer.

In speaking, inspiration is made through the mouth. Inspiration and expiration are not of the same time length. The former is shorter, the latter longer. Trained speakers, actors, radio announcers, singers have very long expiration times. People who are not used to lengthy communication, through living in isolated spots or because of abstinence from communication, have a considerably shorter expiration time. Fatigue, listlessness play a part in respiratory balance.

In singing, respiration is conscious and willed. The chest movements and abdominal movements are carefully balanced. The diaphragm controls the volume of air used, and the best, the most artistic results are obtained through economy, through using the least possible amount of air. One finds this economy of air also used in "artificial" speaking voices, in neurotics who express themselves' in a manneristic way with stress on melodious, "sing-song," talk which requires very little volume of breath.

Activities, emotions and urges are among the involuntary factors that modify breathing. Respiration becomes rapid, irregular, intensified in irritability; shallow and frequent respiration show in embarrassment. Emotional effects on breathing are well known; however, it must be remembered that not only does the actual occurrence of emotions change respiration through a different diaphragmatic activity, but the *recollection* of emotions does the same thing. William B. Faulkner[24] observed the effect on respiration in imaginary situations. Merely suggested anger and pleasure showed under fluoroscopy that the diaphragmatic movements were limited to one-half inch in worry and they expanded to three and one-half inches in joy. These were reflex movements to imaginary situations. It is logical to assume that real emotions would at least have had the same effect if not a greater one. Thus it is understandable that in the swaying back and forth between reality and fantasy in pathological thinking the emotions produced can result in the same respiratory changes that belong to real life situations. This same thing happens in the good actor. He does not "make believe" a certain type of respiration but actually undergoes it by imagining a certain emotion.

Through studies on "inner speech"[25] we learn that to many individuals the thinking of certain words means silent articulation, with the vocal apparatus in position to speak. This again changes respiration. "Inner speech" is inaudible but traceable. Certain words with pleasant or unpleasant associations in themselves do the same thing. In neurotic situations this becomes more pronounced, and associations result in more drastic emotional reactions. The schizophrenic in his frequent hyper-rhythmic motor activities has hyper-rhythmic respiratory patterns. One holds his breath if one smells something bad. This is not necessarily a reflex action to a chemical irritant, but is an acquired response, because whether a particular odor is judged agreeable or disagreeable depends on the cultural period and area in which we live. Patients with olfactory hallucinations undergo respiratory changes, but the haughty person keeps his nose high and he too has characteristically altered respiration.

Here should be mentioned the "lie detector" which registers respiratory changes in connection with blood pressure deviations under emotional influence. Unfortunately, the recordings are made from the chest only, and lack the untapped source of information which could be had were the recordings made from both the chest and the abdomen during respiration. The incongruencies between these two, chest and abdominal breathing, are often characteristic of, for instance, anxiety.

Of course, in voice analysis, just as in medical diagnosis, it is advisable to evaluate a symptom (manner of breathing, in this instance) in relation to other manifestations, and interpret the syndrome, the configuration, rather than an isolated factor. This does not detract in any way from the possible significance of a single symptom within the total picture.

We listen to the following elements and co-ordinations when we analyze respiration in terms of expression:

1. Depth and volume of breathing
2. Frequency of respiration
3. Relation of expiration and inspiration
4. Relation of thoracic versus abdominal functions
5. Relation between the amount of air used and the intended tone
6. Rhythm of respiration

1. *Depth and Volume of Breathing:* A person may breathe deeply or shallowly, use much or little air, depending on his lung capacity, the circumference of his rib cage, and the angle of his ribs to the sternum.

Do depth and volume of breathing express certain basic personality traits? We may safely say that they do, since constitutional development is part of our personality makeup. We know that deep respiration requires far greater muscular effort than does shallow respiration. Breathing also affects the basic chemistry that sustains us. But no matter how much oxygen we breathe in, our metabolism can use only a limited amount. The surplus is wasted and so is the energy used to secure it. Yet the amount, too, has significance. We find that athletic persons and opera singers who do not use a microphone for volume will breathe deeply, as do energetic "go-getters"; while thinkers, speculators, fanciers, "lazy" people will be among the shallow breathers. The Greek runners had to have a special kind of body build to guarantee their endurance in the strenuous activity to which they were trained. Their breathing was shallow, their energy economy was kept at a minimum to ward off fatigue as long as possible. People with great patience and endurance are characterized more by continuous balance of their breathing than by depth or volume.

The basic personality as determined from the constitution includes what Draper[26] so aptly calls the "mosaic of androgyny." Some time ago it was assumed that men breathed one way while women breathed another. We know now that this is not true. But persons who are preponderantly male in their secondary sex characteristics (and thus in their personality) will be likely to breathe deeply and fully because of their wider rib cage, while those with more female components will slide toward the other end of the scale. We must emphasize, however, that the androgynic composition of the individual has no bearing on his potency, reproductive capacity, or sex affinity. And the volume of a person's breathing is not fixed for all time. It varies with activities, circumstances, and emotional states. It is extremely sensitive, and in addition, can be controlled at will. Therefore volume of breathing is an excellent means of expressing emotional symbols. Thus, breathing becomes more than usually shallow in fatigue and in hopelessness. One "holds his breath" in expectation and breaths deeply in release or ecstasy.

2. *Frequency of Respiration:* When analyzing a neurotic voice one needs to find out whether the patient has had training in singing or speaking. Length and frequency of breathing are indicative of training and skill or lack of it. Frequent and shallow inhalations show that the speaker is not used to speaking and may even be averse to it.

One often has an impression of insincerity in listening to high pressure salesmen. This is because one can differentiate between the "canned" sales talk and the unrehearsed story. Smooth breathing technique cannot be simulated in situations where stops for breathing and thinking are indicated.

Frequency of breathing, therefore, may reveal certain basic personality traits (not necessarily constitutional in nature) such as taciturnity, communicativeness and, combined with other features, insincerity. Because of the close, direct connection with metabolism, rapid and frequent breathing indicates over-activity or excitement. The nature of the emotion must be evaluated by its conjunction with other vocal elements. Fear and anxiety create a need for more frequent respiration, while grief and frustration may decrease the frequency.

3. *Relation of Inspiration and Expiration:* The small baby learns to express pleasure and displeasure through the one coordination he controls, breathing. Increased inspiration expresses pleasure, increased exhalation displeasure. *"OOOO-a OOOO-a"* is the effortless rhythm of crying for pleasure, for the sake of activity itself. *"o-AAAA, o-AAAA,"* with muscular stress on exhalation reflects displeasure, rage, pain.

Facing a difficult situation is analogous to facing a distinctly unpleasant one. In this instance speech becomes unbalanced, with quick, audible inspirations and long, forced exhalation, even at times, sighs. Forced expiration also connotes aggression.

While lack of balance between expiration and inspiration may symbolize a variety of emotional meanings, well balanced respiration characterizes an integrated personality. Such a manner of breathing suggests to the listener that the speaker is self-assured, unselfconscious and has control over the immediate situation. The interpretation is rather obvious since such balanced breathing is completely automatic and typical of a relaxed bodily and psychological state.

Diaphragmatic movements are by no means voluntary ones but they are controlled by voluntary movements of the abdominal (mostly lateral) muscle groups. Expiration and consequently phonation are "supported" by these co-ordinations. A tone can be prolonged at will. This is called "appoggio" in singing. In the symptomatology of the "inspiratory voice" (phonation during inspiration) it will be found that this "appoggio," this support, is out of function; the muscle groups remain in inspiratory position. The "in-between" is the so-called quavering voice which is usually connected with a trembling and almost general spastic incoordination. Here the abdominal muscles are retained in a position between inspiration and expiration, as "not finishing" expiration. As a result the diaphragm is held in the same position. In shyness and in fear the support is weak, which shortens the expiratory phase, while in rage a person is often able to sustain the tone to an exaggerated degree.

4. *Relation of Thoracic and Abdominal Function:* The ancient Greeks held that the diaphragm was the center of joy, laughter, grief and weeping, the seat of pride, of self-reliance. Brain and diaphragm were designated by the same word: *phren.* Antique Egyptian and Asiatic sculptures always show deities at the peak of inspiration to imply that animus, breath or spirit is in them.

The diaphragm reacts with sensitivity to emotional moods. In turn its movements alter sounds. Embarrassment upsets the coordination between abdominal muscles, diaphragm, lungs and vocal cords, and as a result an unsteady tone is produced which denotes uncertainty.

While it is an unwarranted oversimplification to say that men breathe with more abdominal participation than women, one may assume that in the mosaic of androgyny, the use of more abdominal function signifies a male component. A "belly laugh" is a very masculine manifestation. It is always hazardous, however, to interpret a single vocal element in this mosaic apart from the influences of other factors, even when it is constitutional in character, because our concepts of male and female expressional traits are necessarily influenced by the mores of our times.

5. *Relation Between the Amount of Air Used and the Intended Tone:* There is a proportion between "the tone intended and the tone produced." In anxiety the character of the tone changes. There may also be an incoordination of the vocal cords which do not always close sufficiently under emotional influence. When a person is apprehensive, he "shrinks." Vocally this means that he tries to keep the tone small. The amount of exhaled air will be bigger than the sound produced. The sound of horror is always breathy. And the word "horror" itself expresses this in the best onomatopoetic way.

The incompletely closed vocal cords make a passage for "wasted" air, "wild air" as Froeschels calls it, which escapes unused for phonation between vocal cords. Fatigue, hopelessness, inhibitions often reveal this symptom. Excitement and expectation show it. We sigh with joy, suck in our breath when surprised, sigh with fatigue, and so on. The particular meaning of the toneless surplus air depends on the vocal syndrome in which it appears.

The most objectionable breathiness, from the listener's point of view, is that of the pseudo-inspired speaker. It is as if this person is under the spell of a colossal semantic mistake; the more he inspires the more "inspired" he will be, and all this audible by long, noisy inhalations.

Whispering is a wide-spread vocal convention often heard in neurotic expression, especially often in schizophrenics. It is the articulated toneless expiration which is intended to be secretive. It is understood that in this case it is not meant as a symptom of organic pathology, as in organic dysphonia. If an individual whispers inordinately, the habit discloses a major character trait. It often interferes with audible inspiration and normal voice. This can be considered an expression of "anal," of retentive personalities. They suck in their breath because they do not want to give it away (in analogy to Abraham's "anal" character[27, 28]).

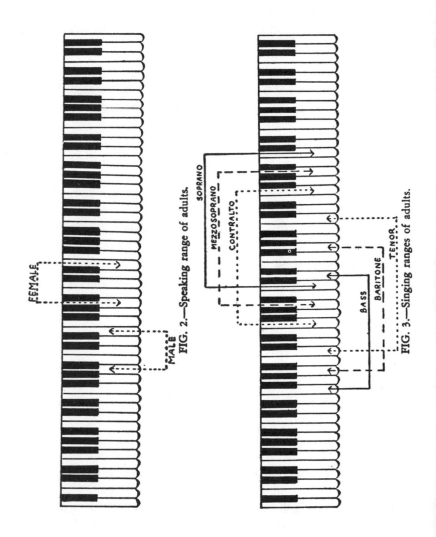

FIG. 2.—Speaking range of adults.

FIG. 3.—Singing ranges of adults.

6. *Rhythm of Respiration:* Rhythm was the means by which the magician in ancient cultures achieved the concentration necessary for the ritual. It was used to exorcise, for direct or remote control, and as a technique of self-hypnosis. Medical hypnosis has proved that by controlling the rhythm of breathing we can create certain emotional states. Our breathing adapts itself to the rhythm of activities when we watch with great concentration. It adapts itself likewise to purely imaginary activities. Studying his respiratory changes while reading poetry and prose himself aided Eduard Sievers,[29] famous linguist and historian of literature, in determining the authenticity of old manuscripts. The respiratory rhythm was changed, therefore the lines were written by a different author. Verses conceived when sitting or walking are influenced by different rhythmic respiratory impulses. The rhythm of breathing changes when certain emotional states are thought of as well as when they are experienced. Again it goes without saying that oscillations between reality and phantasy change respiratory rhythm.

The contagiousness of breathing rhythm becomes most manifest in crowds listening to a speaker. True inspirational speakers have one of two effects: either the listener holds his breath in suspense and feels exhausted when the oration is over, or he is carried along with the speaker's superior breathing technique and comes out feeling elated. But in the mass psychosis of Hitler's giant gatherings, the respiratory rhythm was already conditioned by rolls of drums, which in an hypnotic way prepared the receptability of the crowd: even the breathing function became uniform.

Breathing is shut off by closing the glottis. The earliest syndrome of this mechanism is the breath holding of infants. It is a reaction of infantile rage or attention seeking, and if resentment keeps burning, adult asthma may be its further expression.

RANGE

From the hardly feeble, but limited, beginnings of the infant's first wail, which oscillates around two half-tones, the average individual develops a considerable vocal range by the time he is full grown. Every normal human being has three ranges: the potential, the singing, and the speaking range. The potential range spreads from the highest tone he can emit to the lowest, regardless of the nature or quality of the tone. The singing range includes all the tones, from the lowest to the highest, that have a balanced quality. Oscillograms and kymograms clearly show which tones have such properties. Finally, the speaking range is usually the deepest third of the potential range, although actually many people insist on talking in a range not intended for them. Through persistent use one may achieve an artificial range, but sooner or later the strain will damage the function of his vocal cords. In singing, this forced "superstructure" will lack essential artistic tone quality.

Figures 2 and 3 indicate ranges of adult voices. Women speak about an octave higher than men. Baritone is from C sharp to G sharp, mezzosoprano from c sharp to g sharp. Bass is about two to three tones lower than baritone, and the soprano is two to three tones higher than the mezzosoprano. Contralto is usually one and one-half to two tones lower than the mezzosoprano.

The potential range of a person is determined primarily by physiological factors, such as constitution, heredity, sex. The heredity of high and low voices seems to obey certain laws.[30] Whether or not voice ranges are inherited characteristics has intrigued both students of voice and of genetics. There seems some statistical evidence to substantiate the theory that the potential range is inherited. According to this theory, the soprano voice of the mother and the bass of the father constitute the same hereditary gene *(AA)*, and the tenor of the father corresponds to the alto of the mother *(aa)*. Children of *AA* parents will have soprano and bass voices; offspring of *aa* parents will become tenors and altos. When the parents belong to different categories, the voices of the children will be distributed according to Mendel's ratio (1*A*, 2*Aa*, 1*a*). Individuals with mixed heredity are therefore likely to have baritone and mezzosoprano voices. These statistics refer to the potential singing range of normal adult voices. As to whether the adult will or will not use this potential depends on a great many environmental and pathological factors. The importance of this research is that if the theory is proved correct, our general assumptions on the physiology of vocal change have to be altered. Voice changes then cannot be assumed to be uniform (one octave for boys and a third of this for girls) but the intervals of change are governed by the hereditary patterns.

Certain degenerative processes, such as calcification of the thyroid cartilage and petiolus of the epiglottis, seem to be inherent in the aging process. Voice and age correlate significantly, at least from infancy to maturity. Figure 1 indicates changes in voice range from birth to the age of fifteen.

The fact that the individual has not one but three voice ranges may be less bewildering if one remembers that the speech range of today is only a partial function. In archaic days, when sounds, and not abstract constructions of grammar, were the interpreter of human thoughts and emotions, the complete range of voice was used more freely. Like the infant who lets his vocal powers range to their fullest extent, primitive peoples at the dawn of society used their voices to their hearts' content to express their feelings and reactions. Sensual sound phenomena also preceded syntax. As we ceased to communicate in gestures, imitative sounds, cries of sorrow and jubilation, and acquired, instead, words, our vocal range began to shrink to the point where speech melody is now merely a weazened emotional scale on which rational articulation plays its piece. Only when our controls get out of hand, when we become excited or intoxicated, do we become savages again. We forget our civilized range limitations and the primeval cry can be heard again. Range is the language of emotions, as against articulation, the language of ideas.

Singing is something of a compromise, a willed recall of an echo of the pure satisfaction of primitive vocalization. It is an auto-erotic activity, releasing the tensions built up by our repressions. We sing to express joy and sorrow or because we want to create pleasing sounds; not primarily to elicit admiration.

All civilized people in the world today have narrowed their vocal range for speaking, but within various cultures considerable differences have developed. Among Oriental peoples singing and speaking are distinctly separate functions. Singing is high, speaking is low. There seems to be some geographical differentiation. As we approach the Equator there is a greater frequency of high male and low female voices. Some languages, such as the Romance languages, permit greater vocal freedom than others. An Italian will use a wider range in everyday speech than a Scotsman. Even more interesting is the fact that there are great range variations within the dialects of any one language. In a radius of a few miles in Germany,

France, Italy or Spain one may hear completely different speaking ranges, corresponding to local dialects. The evolution of these dialects has been affected by the languages of the tribes who originally lived there, by invasions and infiltrations or by isolation. Still, if one holds that play on the vocal range is the emotional background to articulation, the vocal differences in dialects assume a complex significance that has not yet been explored.

Indicative of this significance is another cultural phenomenon— the change in vocal fashions. Within our lifetime we have experienced such changes here in the United States. Contrary to Oriental vocal patterns, in Western culture there is no radical difference between the speaking and singing voice. Fashions in singing coincide with fashions in speaking both in the theatre and on the street. If we scan our preferences today, it becomes evident that deep female voices are admired. Most of the ranking actresses in the legitimate theatre have deep voices. In popular singing the higher ranges of the soprano are rare, as they do not appeal to this generation.

These facts are of utmost importance in judging the vocal expression of the neurotic and psychotic. Identification and imitations, introjections, mannerisms and affectations, ideals, as well as rejected patterns do not obey international or eternal laws but are subject to constant change in time and space. The vocal expression of the Italian is normal only within racial and geographic limits, whereas it would be pathological if used by a Scotsman. The pattern accepted as an ideal one by the insecure person varies with these fashions. The same variation in masculinity and feminity of fashions prevails in accepted vocal patterns. Doubtless the present period is often expressed through low female and high male voices. Unless these influences are studied, it is impossible to establish basic ideas about neurotic voices. One has only to see again a movie of the late twenties to discover the normal vocal expression of that period would be considered clearly neurotic today.

Within the geographic limits of temperate countries, soprano and baritone voices are the most common. There are comparatively few contraltos among women and not too many natural tenors among men. But though the potential range of a person's voice is constitutionally given, his speaking range is a matter of training, custom, and personal preference.

Operatic history gives a continuous record of vocal types which represented personality types to their contemporaries. This is the only source which gives us very precise information about prevalent vocal identification during the lifetime of the composer, or what his genius anticipated would follow. Wagner anticipated female emancipation by thirty years in creating the dramatic soprano. Since opera is exaggerated vocal expression, since it is written around the voice and not around the word, one finds a surprising parallelism in its vocal creation and the vocal expression in neurosis. In opera we find the father type, the mother, the non-maternal type, the childish and the child-like voice, the representative of high principles. We find extreme masculinity and extreme feminity expressed by nothing but the voice—on a level which was at one time accepted as characteristic. Opera expresses types in our present-day generation in an inadequate way—screen and playhouse stage are more up-to-date. Opera changes more slowly than popular mores, a cultural lag. Vocal fashions change faster in our day than ever before. More people are more quickly influenced. The phenomenon of experiencing voices through the many sources of vocal reproduction today may be the cause. Today more people are subject to fear because of voices than ever before.

Maternal and paternal voices have characteristic ranges. Authority speaks low. The male teacher, lawyer, judge, the preacher often use a low voice to express authority, utilizing the deepest part of their potential range. Within the authoritative voice there are variations, as for instance, the admonishing range which is the vocal equivalent of the raised index finger. This voice is not only low, but limited in range and restricted in melody. While some languages have narrower ranges than others and while one social group may permit itself more latitude than another, a range that is relatively narrower than customary within the group always indicates inhibitions. The admonishing voice wishes to restrict further the already subdued emotions and tries to manipulate the listener into doing likewise. It is the voice of the Puritan.

Authority carries the connotation of security, especially to children and the weak. In our culture, protectiveness and compassion speak in low, comforting tones and with the chesty ring of sincerity. Teachers and ministers, if they are not the admonishing type, will speak with a fairly wide range and with much chest register. The physician's bedside voice is not too far removed from stereotype, though it has a more restricted melody. Any type of over-compensation or insecurity in authoritative positions can be easily recognized by exaggerations of lowness of voice as well as exaggerated melodious factors. The individual syllable will then acquire a melodious foundation which is out of keeping with the true representation of the word. With regard to range, it becomes evident how ambivalent this dimension is when we note that authority can be expressed both by widening and by shrinking. Widening beyond logic brings the sing-song quality to the voices of many public speakers. Shrinking of range expresses intended matter-of-factness, cutting off any emotional color. It is found in the authoritative utterances of Army personages in high position who want to concentrate on strictly representative communication without self-expressional modulation. The mathematician wants to disappear as a person behind his science and the Army officer tries to maintain distance from the enlisted men by not giving any personal touch to his words. It is easily evident that both these factors will become the expression of over-compensation in neurosis. Some emotions carry with them the reflex action of shrinking. The voice, too, shrinks in range as well as in volume.

One of the known symptoms of hysteria is illogical emotional impact in speaking or emotions expressed by the voice that are contrary to the content. The patient will say something quite trivial in an elated or aggressive voice. Content and voice are therefore disconnected. An inebriated person may lose his inhibitions and his range will become wider and wider until it literally gets out of control and he utters merely low mumblings or high, whining sounds. Enthusiasm and joy break through the limitations of conventional speech and will play on a wide range. Over-emotional and dramatized expression has acquired a new standard pattern which is daily demonstrated to the radio listener in commercials, with the result that it is closer to hysteria than to genuine enthusiasm. Hypocrites and pseudo-benefactors often betray themselves by using a range that is inappropriate to the content. Whereas in our culture use of the lowest third of the potential range is used in normal communication, the Prussian junker and the German Army Officer speak in a highpitched nasal voice. The German man on the street will place the owner of such a voice infallibly in the proper class. But instead of describing this voice as noble, as would the Chinese, the man on the street in Germany will be inclined to call it arrogant.

REGISTER

The term register has been borrowed from the organ, an instrument made to emit the same notes in various ways. As applied to the human voice, register refers to a physical acoustic event which results from an energetic change within the muscular coordination of the vocal cords. How registers function may be seen with the stroboscope, unfortunately under the unnatural conditions obtained during mirror laryngoscopy. In singing from the highest tone possible down to the lowest, the untrained singer first passes a sequence of tones which seems unified. Then he comes to a "node," a switching point, from which he continues with a sequence of tones of a different character. Then he again reaches another "node," and switches to the lowest third of the range produced in a specific tone quality. The trained singer does not reveal these nodes, since he has learned to unify the head-, the mixed, and the chest-register.

While one register prevails, there is no change in the shape of the glottis and the overtones remain the same. The highest is the head-register, the lowest the chest-register. The one in the middle consists of a mixture of both and is therefore called "mixed voice" or mixed register. This is used in normal speaking; it is a well-balanced co-ordination of the width of vocal cords. When high tones are sung by men in head register or "falsetto," a small opening remains between the cords. Vibrations then occur more in the marginal part of the cord, toward the glottis.

Otto Iro[31] has a picturesque way of describing the function of registers. He calls the chest function "earth" and the head function "water." If the two are mixed, the result is "clay." The more water from the head register, the thinner, the more flexible the clay. The more earth, the thicker the clay mixture. This is an excellent analogy to remember, particularly since voices are not classified simply as head, chest, or mixed voices, but are differentiated according to the dominance of one or the other register in the *voce mista,* the unified product. Singers as well as speakers may speak with either more head or more chest function. The more watery clay is termed a lyric voice and the earthy mixture, a dramatic voice.

The term register has been used exclusively for singing where head register in men is called falsetto. A tenor singing falsetto is judged effeminate, or humorous, today and is not accepted as a serious artist. Eighty years ago he could use as much falsetto as he wished and two hundred years ago falsetto singers were considered the exponents of the highest singing art, especially in Spain and Italy. This shows how our aesthetic concepts change in keeping with the prevailing cultural patterns and fashions. Since the head register is produced more internally and the chest register more externally in the vocal cords, we can say that mixed registers as we use them in conversational voice are produced by complete co-ordination of the whole width of the vocal cords. Isolated use of chest register was artistically heard last by the bassos in the Don Cossack Chorus, whose pure chest tones sounded like church bells. It is easily understandable that by using isolated head registers a high voice can be produced which is similar to the high voice which would result from an infantile larynx. The normal adult male larynx produces through this head register a voice which is similar to the voice of the same individual before mutation, while his larynx still had infantile measurements. This fact in itself explains that in fixation to infantile patterns or in regression into childhood the use of this isolated head register is a perfect instrument to simulate childhood situations. If, on the other hand, an individual has the subconscious urge to express through his voice how masculine he is or to what degree he represents father, he can lower his voice only to a certain degree by using the full width of vocal cords. However, by increased use of chest register he is able to lower considerably more, but with detriment to his vocal cords. More important than stressing the use of one or the other registers is the so-called divergence of registers. This concept was introduced into the analysis of the singing voice by Otto Iro. It has not been applied to the speaking voice, where it probably plays a much more important part. With regard to the normal personality, one can say that balanced use of registers expresses a balanced personality with regard to a successful identification. It seems that divergence of registers or the functional inability to co-ordinate registers always expresses conflict in identification. It is an almost quantitative device in the analysis and evaluation of these problems. Two condensed case histories will illustrate these phenomena.

A twenty-five-year-old patient spoke in a high, childlike voice which caused him great embarrassment. He had completely normal vocal chords adequate to produce a healthy baritone and he could actually sing baritone. But he persisted in speaking in falsetto. Another patient, a young lawyer, complained of chronic hoarseness. He used in his voice production an over-amount of chest register. The young lawyer had a prominent father who played a leading role in the country's life and his son had a high ideal to live up to. Hence the forced tone to create an illusion which would hide the lack of success in identification with the father image. Similarly the persistent falsetto of the other patient could be traced to holding on to his mother's apron strings.

Adolescence for both these young men was defeat instead of victory, a rejection of the father, a clinging to the past. In both cases they had to retrace the steps, relearn their lesson in young manhood. Both solved their voice problems within a comparatively short time.

In the early Twenties there developed a new interest in the relation between human physique and personality. Kretschmer[32] and later Sheldon[33] developed many new theories in this field. However, this literature neglected voice and its relation to constitutional types completely. Typing became almost an obsession and new anthropological measuring devices were applied. One factor was neglected: that these types were instinctively used on the operatic stage.[34] For a long time one spoke about the lyric voice in contrast to the dramatic one and one accepted on the stage these voice characters as representative of completely different personality types which were very closely defined. What was not known was the fact that not only the singing voice but the speaking voice as well enveloped the same factors. To use terms describing human constitution we can make the following statement: the voices of different constitutional types are characterized by different proportions in the amount of head and chest registers which together form the mixed voice.[35] The schizoid type has a more prevalent head register. The cycloid or pyknic type has increased chest register within the register mixture. Increased head register means lyrical in the field of singing. Increased chest register means dramatic. The concluding chapter will demonstrate how schizophrenics separate these registers into two different voice patterns which they can use alternately.

RESONANCE

Resonators for the voice are in the chest, the pharynx, the mouth and the naso-pharynx, the nose, the nasal sinuses and in Morgagni's ventricles. These constitute the equipment of the human voice to make itself heard. Low tones are just that; they receive their resonance low in the chest. The high tones find their resonator in a high spot in mouth, nose or naso-pharynx. This is why resonance and register, two completely different functions in the process of voice production, are so often confused with one another. In speech the oral and nasal cavities play the major part. Humidity and the lack of it influence the resonating potentials of the tissues. The soft palate is solely responsible for the gliding change from mouth to nose or naso-pharynx. It acts as a retractable closure, somewhat like an overhead garage door, separating or uniting the oral and nasal cavities (Fig. 4). People who pronounce with great care and exactness usually have an active palate, as is true of persons whose voice reflects a variety of emotions and moods. "Sloppiness" is not confined to shuffling gait; nasal draw belongs in the picture. It is fashionable with teen-agers to drag the soft palate in the same way they drag their feet. People living in warmer climates have a tendency to avoid muscular exertion; hence at least a partial cause for

the difference between standard English and German and the variations of the southern dialects of these languages. While considerable tenseness of palate activity may be observed in the former, the
southern variations show a decided decrease of movement and thus
a resulting increase in nasality. Other cultural traits may be attributed to this controllable soft palate action. As noted before, the
Chinese and Japanese, using head register and high tones for
artistic expression, such as singing and recitation, also express "higher
emotions" in a nasal tone comparable again to the haughty nasality
of the Prussion Junker officers.

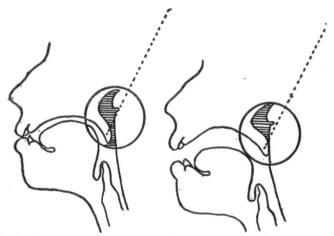

FIG. 4.—Functioning of the soft palate. Mechanism of nasal resonance: (a)
open, nasal tone; (b) closed, oral tone.

But resonance is also subject to involuntary emotions and urges.
The nasal mucous membranes are closely related in function to the
swell bodies of the sex organs, but the nasal turbinates seem to be
more sensitive. They are affected by many emotions other than sex
urge. Studies by Thomas H. Holmes and his associates[36] seem to
indicate that functional changes of the nose accompanying sexual
activity, menstruation, and pregnancy depend on the individual's
psychological and emotional responses to the total situation more
than to the amount of sex hormones. In these studies by Holmes,

hypo- and hyperfunctions of nasal structures under the influence of emotions were well observed from intensely swollen to dry and shrunken mucous membranes. However, neither they nor some of the older authors, such as Koblank,[37, 38] made the obvious inference that these changes must necessarily be reflected in the voice and that therefore voice would disclose particular conditions even before nasal examinations or psychological tests were applied. Since nasal resonance depends on resonator space and on the conditions, especially humidity, of the tissues, both the degree of swelling and the amount of discharge will affect the voice. It is important to state that the experiments for nasal swelling have had the same results which Faulkner showed for the diaphragm; namely, that the recollection of emotional states has an affect similar to the actual situation. This is of great importance in studying the voice of the neurotic who in his intensified emotional recollections will reveal many vocal symptoms which actually mirror the real dramatic situation. Changes in moods and feelings measurably affect respiration and nasal resonance in the average person. To the singer, the actor, or the professional speaker, this presents a very real problem. Stage fright can produce swelling of the nasal mucous membrane, inhibiting resonance, which will resemble a cold. This symptom will be described in a later chapter on neurosis of the singer.

The voice of an ascetic person is literally dry. The tone will always reveal the lack of cushioning and the lack of moisture. Asceticism is a psychological state resulting from hyperfunction of certain glands or in a psychosomatic way controlling these functions. Since all bodies capable of swelling act interconnectedly, it is obvious that the membranes of the nose will also be reduced in bulk and moisture. A person who tries to be an ascetic and has stormy conflicts does not talk with the voice of an ascetic. The nose becomes a truer witness to our real emotional situations than our words or our intentions.

If situations such as pregnancy, intercourse, or menstruation are resented or feared, the conflict will again find vocal expression. At this time it is not known whether intense change of voice with marked swelling of the nasal mucous membranes during pregnancy can be explained by emotional factors, such as resentment of the situation. It is well known that many singers sing their best during menstruation, whereas others complain of such marked nasal swelling that singing becomes impossible. Whether the former accept the situation and the latter resent it is unknown, but the question could well be investigated.

In true fear situations, mucous membranes become dry and the turbinates shrink. Clinical experience shows dry vocal cords and closed salivary glands. Therefore the voice sounds extremely oral, without the warming touch of nasal resonance. The expression of closeness in love shows marked participation of nasal resonance; whereas desire for distance, the various degrees in the urge to be left alone, is expressed by complete elimination of nasal resonance with exclusive use of resonance spaces within the mouth cavity. This oral voice can therefore be found in schizophrenics who, although they talk constantly, do so in monologues without any intention or desire for real communication.

Another mechanical factor in resonance should not be neglected. Facial expressions influence both articulation and tone. An overly tense mouth and jaw often express forced determination and energy, usually as overcompensation. Inhibitions of various types interfere with releasing control of facial muscles. This results in interference of tone by changing oral resonance.

RHYTHM

Rhythm is one of the most sensitive dimensions. Its changes are audible and measurable under different emotions, and each individual has his own individual rhythm. There is nothing static about rhythm. Rhythm is movement, it is tension and release, and it is periodicity. Perhaps the best definition of rhythm for our purposes is organization of movement, the perception of which is principally an intellectual act (Dom Joseph[39]). Sensation becomes experience only through repetition. The baby's lalling is a pleasurable, unconscious, involuntary repetition of oral movements resulting in sound production. It is maximum result with a minimum expenditure of energy. Labial play is repeated because the pleasure comes with less exertion than it would by changing to other muscle movements. At the same time, this duplication conditions the brain centers to: (a) perceiving the sound; (b) the ability to reproduce later the movements, and consequently the sound, at will; (c) connecting the sound with other sensations and perceptions. This would be impossible without rhythmical repetition.

We assimilate by making helpful processes automatic and by suppressing all disturbing processes. This is habit formation, and its main source is rhythm. All our automatic processes, breathing, walking, talking, have rhythm. According to Kafka, all sensory experiences, especially sound, evoke motor reactions, which are rhythmically organized.[40]

The human voice has an inevitable rhythmic beat and all language is inescapably cadenced. Even the rhythms of our internal processes modify each other and sometimes come into conflict, as for example when the pulse beat interferes with vocalization, injecting a tremolo into a prolonged sound.[41]

Because of the constant change in environment as well as within the human being, the periodicity of rhythm in living things cannot be quantitatively exact. Like the waves of the ocean which are similar but never the same, physiological rhythm is irregular. Regular rhythm lacks life. It is typical of the machine, of artificiality, of the beat of attempted mechanical perfection.

Although we are far from fully understanding the meaning of rhythm, one recognizes it as an essential element of human physiology and psychology. Rhythm of speech, our common vocal expression, must in some way reflect both our personality and our pathology. When the beat of our lower physiological processes intrudes on our speech rhythm, it indicates deterioration of the higher centers. Because of the complexity of the rhythms of internal physiological processes and the infinite variability of the human species, no two persons are born with the same constitutional rhythm pattern. This innate pattern is greatly modified by the time one reaches maturity. External rhythms impinge on the individual; one acquires new rhythms by the learning process; we come into conflict with rhythms which are alien to us.

To understand the meaning of rhythm one must trace its archaic evolution, as music and rhythm preceded the use of words. Magic, religion, science and the "word," the name of a thing, are closely interwoven. The close connection of chant and magic is suggested by the very word "enchantment." Rhythmic expression is a central feature in all evocation. Rhythm in ancient magic had three roles: to exercise remote control of the force to be subjugated by symbolic gesture and repeated invocations of its name, to create the concentration necessary for magic ritual, and to submerge the magician into a state of even greater antiquity where he could explore the unconscious for "inner voices," racial memories, Urgefühl. Sometimes rhythm helped to achieve actual control through hypnosis, self-hypnosis, and practices similar to present-day yoga. It is evident that in rhythm we face a dimension which, more than any other, reveals qualities reaching far back to the primary expressions of mankind.

In the development of the individual, rhythm is the one experience which the newborn brings with him into the world. This prenatal experience enables the infant to assimilate the sensations which come to him after birth. The individual rhythmic pattern is modified by external and internal influences, not the least of which is volition. But as soon as volition and vigilance relax, the primary rhythm of the individual breaks through the superstructure. Some people doodle when they daydream, others drum on the table. Biological rhythm, the original "life force," the magic power, has ascended from the unconscious and has taken hold of the relaxed individual.

Rhythmic repetition of an event helps the individual to retain the original coordination with which he first received the stimulus, instead of his having to adapt to a new and different coordination. For example, the ear becomes used to a sound heard repeatedly. It will assume the necessary coordination easily and the release that comes with the realization of expectation will be pleasurable. A new sound pattern means a new coordination, which in turn means effort, and therefore in a sense, pain. This is the reason why unfamiliar voices are apt to make children cry. Any new stimulus creates tension and expectation. If the release is delayed too long, the rhythm is disturbed. Stimulus is piled upon stimulus without release and creates blocks and frustrations. If on the other hand, the sequence between expectation and release is too short, the individual cannot perceive it and therefore the experience will not exist in his consciousness; or, if it does, it will leave him unsatisfied. Normal rhythm is always a source of pleasure because of the release of tension and this is clearly evident in the expression of the normal child. During adolescence a change in individual expressional rhythm breaks through the vocal superstructure imposed by education and group association. But the rhythmic pattern has not yet crystalized. The author found this consistently true in the sixty-odd blind listening tests of adolescents' voices conducted at the Adolescent Growth Study, Institute of Child Welfare, University of California (see Introduction). The individual rhythm that was so marked in pre-school age must be developed anew when school influences have worn off. Since in adolescence the development is still fluid, the individual has not yet made a decision about his future permanent self—the rhythmic features of his voice are indistinct and variable.

Rhythm is an ambivalent phenomenon. More rhythm does not mean necessarily better rhythm, nor does less rhythm mean worse. Our rhythmic needs vary greatly both individually and socially. With increasing affect, speech becomes more rhythmic. Growing excitement produces hyper-rhythm.

Contending that vocal dynamics express psychodynamics, we see that normal rhythm is the composite of:

1) The individual's biological rhythm pattern
2) The rhythm of the language which serves as a medium and which had to be learned
3) The understanding of the meaning inherent in the utterance

As Stockert[44] explains it: rhythm is the physiognomy of speech, modified by elements which express the momentary affect situation. The higher the potential perceptiveness of the individual, the more pronouncd the modulation of his expressiveness. The less his faculty for perceiving, the more uniform and monotonous is his rhythm of speech.

The introvert's speech rhythm will be toned down because he has no desire to convey appeal, while the extrovert, who wants to communicate and to make an impression and see the effect, will intensify the rhythmic elements of speech.

Hitler's voice was hyper-rhythmic. It had a drumming quality. He repeated the same words over and over again; one may say that he made the content rhythmic, and his emphasis was a dynamic stress. His way of speaking was almost "staccato," without any legato element. The voice even more than the content generated mass-hypnosis.

In contrast, the late President F. D. Roosevelt's voice had a swinging melody which served to underline content. The rhythm was "easy," a mere framework to help assimilate what he had to say. His voice had an outgoing quality, meeting halfway the listener's own rhythmic needs.

Rhythm and rhythmic patterns are modified constantly, more or less subtly, because of the constant change in the "affect situation." Panic will remove the inhibitory factors, and speech, like movements, will be "all rush and rescue, and hurry away." Shock may create a spasm which momentarily freezes the voice, while enthusiasm may exaggerate itself into hyper-rhythmic college cheers or the Sieg-Heil cries of the Nazis.

The Ambivalence of Rhythm in Pathology: In certain cases of post-encephalitic disorders, the speech impulse remains intact. The person wishes to express himself, he has the language intact, so to say, in his brain, but his motor reactions are so delayed as to make him seem unresponsive. In other cases, the speech impulse is also exhausted. It is as if in one case the breakes were binding, whereas in the other fuel is lacking too. But in neither of these cases is speech rhythm the central focus of the disorder.

The distinguishing characteristic of human speech as compared to animal communication is the use of symbols for the representation of objects and concepts and the expression of relationships. This latter is inherent even in the simplest human utterances. Language has to be learned and meaningful dynamics learned with it. The fundamental nature of speech dynamics is illustrated in the jumbled "word salad" of certain mentally ill patients, in which, the intonation of perfectly meaningful sentences may be brought forth, indicating that some thought Gestalt, some relational judgment persists in the mind. On the other hand, there are illnesses where the centers of thought formation are affected or blocked, and in these cases accentuation and melody will subside into monotone, and rhythm will not follow the requirements of the language medium. For example, certain schizophrenic patients express a tendency to alliteration and will stress every R or P in what they say, until they give the impression of deliberately filling their utterances with words composed of R's and P's. Here again the ambivalence of rhythm is noticeable; rhythm is destroyed in the sense that it does not correspond to the rhythm of the language medium, but is exaggerated to the extent of machine-like timing by reiterations and by the stressing of short and long syllables. It was described by Faust[43] as withdrawal of acute attention and volition behind biological drives, a degenerative symptom.

There is much debate about the kinship of schizophrenic and infantile speech. In both, rhythm and reiteration prevail. Mothers who bring their feeble-minded children to the speech clinic will often hopefully remark, "You should see how well my little girl dances." And so she does, but not because she is musical or has an understanding of what she hears. Her reaction to rhythm is pronounced and so is her preference for rhythmic behavior. But her development stopped at a lower rhythmic level than is needed for acquiring speech. Schizophrenics may say senseless rhythmic sentences over and over again for months or years and combine this with seemingly meaningless rhythmic gestures. This can be a regression to archaic infantile patterns, in which words, language, communication have lost meaning, but rhythm has not. However, the highly complex distortions of schizophrenic rhythmic behavior are probably fundamentally different from infantile phases of development. We are not sure whether we face phylogenetic or ontogenetic regressive patterns.

Speech on its ultimate, refined level must have universal semantic validity at least within the immediate group, and so also must speech rhythm. Along with this, similar affect values must be attached to the rhythmic element of dynamics by members of the normal group. It is clearly understood that, within normal limits, as higher affect content increases the rhythm of speech and gives us universally enjoyable poetry, so the lower affect content produces decreased but still understandable rhythm. On the pathological level the discrepancies in the semantic values attached to rhythm create a gulf between the normal and the sick which is hard to bridge. Just as the English lady will be repulsed and possibly frightened by the rapid and dynamic word-fire of a well-meaning Sicilian, the vocal dynamics of some demented people will create a wrong reaction, even in the attending physician. One hopes that dynamic psychiatry will succeed in bridging the gulf to create mutual understanding.

CHAPTER IV

Other Acoustic Dimensions and Significant Features of Voice

MELODY

VOICE WITHOUT MELODY is truly meaningless. Even an involuntary cry of pain has melody. Long before articulated sound became the standard means of communication among human beings, vocalization had to be eloquent. The infant's commanding cries and piteous wails bear witness to this expressiveness.

Children learn to speak in simple sentences. Even the simplest grammatical constructions, such as "gim-me" or "bye-bye," have specific meanings indicated by appropriate melodies, and the child learns these along with articulation. Sometimes the articulation will still be poor while the melody makes the meaning entirely understandable.

As the brain cortex develops and becomes capable of more complex functioning, thoughts are logically arranged on the subconscious level in their totality before being expressed vocally. If this were not so, how could one come out spontaneously with the proper sentence formations and synchronized melody? This capacity to anticipate what will follow the word just spoken, to deliver the finished thought vocally without conscious rehearsal, is a high cortical achievement. William James was the first to call attention to the fact that a person reading aloud must, so to speak, sense at the very beginning of the sentence what is to follow; otherwise he could not give it a meaningful melody.

Since writing can indicate only some of the broadest directions of the dynamics of thought, with symbols such as the period and question mark, and is not adapted to expressing the finer nuances of meaning, the accomplishment of reading aloud an unfamiliar text seems even more remarkable. Not only must the reader expect the general content of what follows, but he also must sense the intent of the writer; for example, flattery, irony or doubt.

The function of melody is dramatically shown by patients with sensory aphasia. Sometimes the patient is not able to say more than one word. Still, from senseless chatter, one can unfailingly tell whether the patient is angry or complaining, whether he is greeting someone or wants to go to the bathroom. The intent, but not the content, is communicated by nothing but the melody.

Certain words are impregnated with emotions. These may vary according to cultures, but each culture has a number of such "loaded" words. For us "God," "death," "peace" have intrinsic values. A phrase-mongering orator may elicit emotional responses from his audience with skillful manipulation of loaded words. Taboo will also give certain words a special feeling and thus a special melody. To evoke the name of Jesus in Italian is a simple imprecation, delivered freely and frequently by pious and impious alike, whereas in English it is blasphemy and thus bears corresponding vocal marks. In American-English "bloody" is a matter-of-fact descriptive word without any special coloring. In Britain it can get into print only by elision and stigmatizes speech as uncouth. Personal complexes and taboos affect speech melody, and individual vocal stereotypes can point to the crux of many a nervous problem.

Speech melody is determined first by the grammatical structure of a sentence or, more precisely, by the meaning which underlies the grammatical structure, and secondly, by the inherent emotional value of certain expressions. It also carries the marks of the speaker's moods and attitudes.

Since it is clear how melody of speech is affected by any change of affects and emotions, the diagnostic value of this dimension in neurotic conditions becomes evident.

Melody, in speaking and in singing, can be isolated from other vocal elements. It can be scored, measured and reproduced. Every language and every dialect sings in its own way. The unfading success of the traditional vaudeville act in which the actor speaks gobbledgook in any number of languages is based on the appreciation of this endemic melody. We may not understand what a person says, but we recognize the language.

In any one language, the sentence is a sequence of pitches resulting in an organized musical structure. The voice rests only occasionally on one note. It glides continuously from one tone to another, up and down, around a basic pitch. When we write down the musical score of a particular sentence, we indicate merely the points between which the voice glides in continuous motion. Other, more exact, recordings of speech melody, such as those made with a kymograph, show this continuity clearly, and it can also be perceived by ear if the ear is keen and is trained in auditive observation.

Melody is greatly affected by the relationship between speaker and listener. For example, in the following conversation: "Do you know whom I met yesterday?" "No.", the answer, "No," if given in a low, falling tone implies lack of interest or even rebuke. On the other hand, if the inflection is rising, it is an invitation to a continued conversation.

Unless the speaker has unusual restraint and self-control, his moods will be mirrored in his melody. For example, to the question "How are you?" the standard answer is "Fine, thanks!" In a high pitch it means, "I really feel fine, thank you." In a low or falling pitch it implies dissatisfaction with the state of one's health. Certain occupations seem to develop an indigenous speech melody. That is why it is so easy to parody a politician, a teacher, a minister. It is as if the individual wished to hide his particular shortcomings behind the mask of a socially approved stereotyped score. Because of this lack of genuineness, parody and original are hardly distinguishable. These stereotypes can be found under many neurotic disguises. When it is so easy to copy, it will become the imitated pattern in introjection, in "borrowed" expression of the wish-dream ideal. It will become uniformity, the accepted pattern of groups, orders, fraternities, gangs. Whoever wants to "belong" and feels he is still outside will first accept this melodious pattern.

Melody is far more complicated in its expressional manifestations than are either range or register. It operates on the keyboard of the range and uses registers (and rhythm and volume) to paint an emotional background for the story. It is therefore a complex phenomenon that has to be understood by evaluation of its elements. Moods are expressed in musical keys. Flaubert, the French poet and novelist, spoke his poems aloud both in major and minor before writing them down. His poems are distinguished by their melodiousness. Sad and mellow moods are supposed to be associated with the minor keys and briskness with majors. Helmholtz[42] attributes the melancholy effect of minor chords to a slight dissonance which is not present in the majors. It seems that the emotional effects in vocal music are more defined than in instrumental music (Schoen[45]). It is hard to explain why primitive tribes did not use minor keys to express sadness but sang in minor keys on most occasions, including victory celebrations. Children use more minor keys. A theory has been established that using minor requires less muscular exertion. This phenomenon can be applied in the analysis of the depressed voice. One often hears marked minor key with a tendency to lower the pitch. Each impulse to lower is accompanied by decrease in intensity. It is as if the strain of maintaining a higher pitch is too much for the patient. Again the minor key would prevent greater strain.

When an orator approaches the end of his speech, the audience anticipates it through the key and pitch of his words more than through content: this is somewhat similar to the return to C major in music, which can indicate the festive final cords. It means finality, accomplished fact, in speech as well as in music. How different is this end in the neurotic! Indecision, fear, anxiety, guilt do not permit the "C major" which is combined with a definite lowering of the last syllable meaning the end of a declarative sentence. A statement is accepted as such only if the last syllable has this "true ring of conviction"; analytically speaking, the lowest tone in the sentence with increased chest register. Under anxiety, the patient does not commit himself to this finality. Figuratively he keeps the door open by not lowering final syllables, and immediately the statement assumes the melody of a question: rising melody at the end of a sentence, in the last syllable of a word, or in the last vowel in monsyllables. The width of the interval indicates the emotional meaning, the curiosity.

It is not only the pitch of one syllable that may fall and rise but so may also the melody of an entire word, clause, or statement. A declining melody, particularly if it is repeated regularly, connotes depression. A classic example of this is the famous speech of Edward VIII in which he abdicated for the "Woman I love."

Perhaps the greatest variability in melody is found in its intervals—the difference between pitches of individual syllables. Wide intervals characterize excitement, including excitement from toxic influences such as alcohol and drugs. All the manic emotions are channeled through comparatively large intervals. In operatic music one hears a parallel evidence: in recitativo the small intervals represent facts, thought, remarks. In arias the large intervals express feelings.

The ambivalence of melodious expression must guide the analyst in his evaluation. Small intervals can mean modesty and orderly realism. But the voice as well may be utilitarian, puritanistic, secretive and cold. A voice that uses large intervals freely and frequently is expressive of emotions, genuine or simulated, which in other words means that the person is rich in feelings or that he has the power of representation or both. On the negative side, large intervals may mean pomposity, exaggeration, or lack of emotional balance.

If the melody of depression is constant in a voice, the person reveals a pathological symptom. Adaptability to situations will be expressed through a flexible voice. Stiffness suggests resistance to influence, stubbornness or reserve.

INTENSITY; SPEED

Speech melody is an organic structure with dynamic accents of volume and speed modifications. While variations in pitch carry the specific meaning, and to a certain extent the emotional undertones, of the conveyed thought, changes in intensity underline importance, focus attention, and thus express appeal. Intensity modulations are important elements of vocal communication. The stressed word is usually louder and higher and longer. Intensity changes in direct relation with the pitch.

The intensified consonant is connected with the preceding or following vowel. No real consonant can be increased in volume by itself. Intensities can be measured by various means and can be described in graphic form. The ear, however, is perfectly adequate to tell us whether someone talks loudly or softly, as well as what elements of speech are dynamically underscored. The intensity of an entire sentence may be increased or a single word or single syllable may be stressed.

Intensity changes must be evaluated relatively rather than absolutely. In a sentence shouted in great excitement there still will be some more distinct accent, focusing attention on the central core of the exclamation. A whispered sentence may include a softly accented word, but this will express a relative increase in volume and thus a meaningful stress. "Emphasis" designates the increased intensity of a sentence while "accent" places stress on a word or syllable.

The dynamics of speech are learned. When the nervous system of the baby attains the capacity to feel pain, his first shout in reaction to pain will impregnate that particular sound, dynamics and all, with the meaning of pain for him. Intensity, when used in a meaningful way, even in the most primitive of meanings, is part of an acquired pattern.

The child learns intonation and accentuation together with the meaning of a concept. The first words are uttered with a purely rhythmical stress, evolved from repetition. But the child quickly learns the difference between "Mommy, *come!*" and "*Mommy* come!" Both are commands but they have specific meanings expressed by the accent.

Because stress is a learned quality, it is subject to many environmental influences, and is a sensitive measure of them. Lack of education can be easily detected from the mispronunciation of words. But intensity also discloses constitutional and pathological conditions. Emphasis and accentuation clarify meaning, focus thought, and help make the dispersed elements of thought into an organic whole. The mentally defective will often speak with differentiation of intensity or with confused accents.

Because of all the various dynamic elements intensity is most easily perceived, it is the most easily misinterpreted. Germans speaking English often sound "arrogant" to the American ear. Meeting a "foreigner" necessitates broad experiences and an open mind to avoid the archaic fear reaction. This is the reason most inexperienced people in conversation with foreigners raise their voices instead of pronouncing more carefully. They yell away the evil spirits.

According to Stockert, accentuation is a complex reactive adjustment to stimuli received from external reality. In other words, what we say makes sense. When this meaningful rhythm subsides, giving way to a mere repeating beat, "perceptivity and reacting potentiality to external stimuli are disturbed." Attention and volition withdraw, and the uniform rhythm of fundamental biological processes takes over. Rhythmically accentuated speech at the expense of meaning, therefore, is a pathological symptom of degenerative character. It can be found in neurosis as well as in psychosis.

Intensity is ambivalent. In ordinary speech, greater volume as well as higher pitch are used to accent the appropiate syllable in a word. Actually, the extent of the variation from the norm and not the direction of the change is important. Whispering can center attention on a word just as much as shouting, if the remainder of the sentence is spoken in a normal tone of voice. The dynamics of accents become more pronounced in excitement, when one is more emotional or more eager to explain something. As to whether one lowers or raises his voice to achieve the effect depends on the occasion, personality, training, nationality and many psychological factors.

Intensity is a manifestation of basic psychological energies. On the positive end of the ambivalent scale, increased loudness expresses vitality, creativeness and aggressiveness. On the negative end it can mean brutality, gross sensuality, and intemperance. Strong urges and impulses heighten all dynamic expressional processes. The physician often infers from their intensities the cultural level of patients during a first office visit. Intensity, for the purposes of interpretation, must be subdivided into volume and stress. Volume is easily measured by ear.

What emotional symbols are expressed through these intensities? Anger, if given free play, will roar. But since civilizations have disapproved of these displays, anger has learned to speak without such volume. Tender feelings are supposed to float on soft notes, but so do deception and seduction. Soothing and highly manipulative voices, such as those used in hypnosis, must also speak softly, since it is this quality, together with rhythmic repetition, that wields the decisive influence. Self-dramatization does not depend on magnitude but rather on the variation of volume.

Short intensity, best described by "yapping," expresses the kind of defensive aggressiveness that jabs and runs, or its playful counterpart, coyness. Joviality, hail-fellow-well-met aggressiveness, is symbolized by over-all loudness of the voice, as is the exhibitionism of the "life of the party." But loudness is intrinsic also in the voice of the frustrated shrew.

These last examples indicate that habitual use of vocal emotional symbols stamps a personality with a "trait." But loudness is often misleading in evaluation, much like fatness which has been confused with friendliness and honesty even by Shakespeare. Caesar could have been betrayed by a fat man as well as a lean one. A loud voice is not necessarily jovial, nor must it be perpetually angry.

Volume in itself does not yield us the specific nature of the urge or emotion which gave it birth. It is merely a clue to the impact of this urge and the strength of the willed control that it encounters. The anger of a man who speaks softly may be greater than the anger of a man who shouts. Moreover, it may be deadlier, because it is paired with a will that knows how to exercise self-control.

Accents are vocal manifestations of very different psychodynamic forces. They intensify the emotional undertone but do not disclose the nature of emotion. A sense of form may indicate the *l'art pour l'art* aesthetic inclination of a speaker who has no shred of human compassion, or it may indicate the rapture of self-immolation. Musical accent does not denote control or lack of control relative to the forces of urges and drives, but it rather discloses the basic emotional tonus of the personality.

Grammatical accents are learned in childhood. Generally faulty accentuation or lack of accentuation is an obvious symptom of mental deficiency. Variability in intensity is in direct ratio to perceptivity and sensitivity. Still, one should not assign to intensity any specific trait or symbol. The possible exception is the intensification of consonants, which is contrary to the rules of the English language and of many other languages. This is usually a symptom of repressed aggressiveness and often points to vindictiveness and spite. It is akin to stuttering, though a stutterer is usually a less aggressive personality than the one who "spits" his consonants into the listener's face.

SPEED

To understand the essence of intensity and speed of speech one has to know how and why they are produced. The "how" is understandable physiologically. The "why?" can be fairly well answered with regard to intensity, which in its variability is directly related to cortical development. The more highly developed the cortex, the more meaningful and varied is the intensity modulation. An organic relationship between body development and speed is much harder to prove. The feeble-minded person may have difficulties with speaking, but he will not necessarily speak slowly. Some of the fastest talkers are feeble-minded, which does not make fast-talking a pathological or constitutional-pathological sign. Neither does variability of speed mean higher development.

To measure the number of words or phonemas per minute is of little scientific value. One person may speak fast with long pauses, another hardly stops for breath. A third will talk slowly with short pauses or slowly with long pauses. Speech may be "legato" in gradual transition from one tone to another, or "staccato," words pronounced rapidly with frequent separations. Pauses may be at the end of a sentence, between clauses, between words, or within words. Therefore one has to measure not only the duration of phonation but also the length of the pauses between and determine the pattern of how they are related to each other. To compare various speeds, one compares the elements and the composite.

Everyone to whom language or speech presents difficulties will talk slowly. The child will speak slowly when he learns a word, though once he learns it, he will take great pleasure in repeating it rapidly. A child with highly developed pictorial thinking will speak more slowly during the learning process than the one with motor-acoustic imagination because the latter will translate heard sounds quickly into movements and thus into speech.

Not much is known about organic factors which affect speed, but several pathological syndromes include elements that have a bearing on it. Heart and lung diseases and other conditions affecting respiration have symptomatic speech patterns. Often a patient, knowing that his breathing is limited, tries to pack into one breath as much as possible. The result is the characteristic panting fast talk and gasping long pauses of dyspnea. This is typical of patients shortly after surgical procedures causing paralysis of the recurrent nerve. The left vocal cord does not move; however, the right cord guarantees a glottis which is sufficiently wide for respiration. Still the patient talks with marked dyspnea, "as if being choked." This condition causes a typical anxiety which in conversion often prevents the organically normal right cord from moving toward the midline.

Under normal conditions one says it quickly if one really *wants* to say it. Good news, hopeful expectations, lend wings of joy to speech. In contrast, when there is no impulse, through indifference or an impulse slowed down by illness or depression, speech becomes relatively slow. There is no "average" speed of speech. Desire to communicate and inhibitions and obstacles to this impulse cannot be evened out.

Speech lends itself to oral gratification and therefore autoerotic factors will influence tempo. Blessing and curses are pronounced slowly, as if tasted in the mouth. Emotionally loaded words, as mentioned before, are mostly overarticulated, slowly, whereas taboo words—usually short in English—are produced with a quick intensity and a spitting component.

Since vocal dynamics are psychodynamics, speed and changes in speed actually reflect psychic changes. Although some languages lend themselves to faster or slower speed, there is no language that *demands* fast speaking, though some necessitate slower tempi (Hungarian and Finnish demand exact articulation, slowing down the speed).

Each individual has an optimum tempo with which he moves, speaks, and breathes in his sleep. This tempo is the result of his complex physiological rhythms. The expressional significance of speed is twofold: First, it represents this constitutional personality; second, it indicates when purpose alters the vegetative beat. Both the man of action and the dreamer will speed up when circumstances demand it. The pressure of urge or drive may transcend the repressing elements and break through the established conformation.

A fast voice may be expressive or persuasive, or it may be irritable, garrulous, boring. A slow voice may have convincing force or cloying sweetness.

The essential significance of speed is still elusive. One therefore must deal with it pragmatically in relationship with other elements of voice.

PATHOS

There are certain vocal phenomena which, though clearly distinguishable by the trained ear and even perceived by the untrained ear, have as yet defied quantitative analysis. Because of their significance, however, they cannot be omitted in a description of analytical factors.

If on the stage one sees a king with his crown, his purple, his regalia, one does not doubt that he is king. If one listens to the same play over the radio and can identify the king minus regalia, simply from his voice, then one can say that the player has the pathos of a king.

This "something" that expresses in the voice what a person is in his own estimation, and in mine and yours, is pathos. It is the bridge of identification between "I" and "myself" and "I" and "you." It is the threshold of personal expression. It conveys that the king is king to himself and to you and to me. It makes the child wince at the rejection in his mother's voice, regardless of her words. It moves the congregation during a sermon of true conviction even when the minister is a poor orator. If rhythm expresses the relationship between an individual and the outside world, pathos expresses the relationship between the individual and himself, and between himself and society. Its analytical value for the voice of the neurotic is obvious.

It is difficult to pin down the vocal details that create the resulting impression to pathos. There is no norm to pathos. It is as variable as there are societies and personalities. For example, a young girl's voice may disclose deep emotional qualities. A mature woman's voice saturated with equally deep feelings will sound quite differently. The genuineness in one and in the other is related constitutionally and psychologically to the "I" expressed.

The second key feature of pathos can best be explained by another example. Unless one knows Chinese theatre tradition, neither the king nor the hero nor the villian can be identified. Or, if one were to listen today to an exact contemporary recording of a performance of Victorian tragedy with famous actors of that time, one might surmise that the play is satire, even comedy. There is no doubt that the Chinese play has immense meaning to the Chinese audience, and the original performance of the Victorian tragedy met with an enthusiastic reception by the contemporary audience. Expression of genuine feelings must be there. But social relations have changed in the intervening years since the Victorian drama—that bridge between society and the individual is missing for us today. This exemplifies the importance of the "I" and "you" relationship; pathos cannot exist without a common ground of understanding and identification.

Since pathos is the threshold of self-expression, it entails the intensification of all normal vocal elements particular to a personality. In other words, an emotion that oversteps the breaking point and makes a shrieking maniac of an otherwise quiet, self-possessed person is not pathos and it does not evoke "sympathy." It evokes fear or disgust or restraining action. The threshold that has been crossed is not that of personality expression but of sanity. The intensification of pathos always stays within the normal limits of vocal expression; for this very reason pathos is ambivalent.

A minus or a plus sign must be put before pathos to show that it intensifies largeness into even larger and smallness into even less. To indulge in a somewhat oversimplified psychoanalytical analogy: In the mouth of an "oral" personality, an outgoing, questing, buccaneer, an understatement would be just as out of place as would a gross exaggeration coming from the lips of an "anal" personality, a cautious, reserved, frugal man. The former could indulge quite naturally in colorful vocal exaggerations, while the latter would express pathos by increased reserve in his voice. A very similar manifestation has been observed in handwriting by Klages[46] and Saudek.[47] The exaggeration of large movements into larger and small movements into yet smaller have equal significance.

In our Western culture two important vocal features seem to reveal pathos, although they do not determine it completely. The first is the pitch of the last syllable and the second is the size of the intervals and their directional movement.

Question, exclamation, doubt, suspicion, fear, confidence all of these tugging and pulling forces between the "I" and "you" seem to come to a climax at the end of the spoken thought. Raised pitch, powered pitch, intensification, softening, descending to the lowest pitch, or holding the level can make the last syllable into a sharp sword or a velvet touch. This is the part of the sentence that hits or hurts or soothes. It can be an outstretched hand or a kicking foot. It may express appeal or rejection.

The intervals and their movements from low to high, or high to low, are the emotional keyboard of our speech. Pathos, being the reflection of our emotional profile, is mirrored in the musical intervals. Pathos of pride, pathos of feeling, pathos of will, all compulsive expressions of emotions, must use this channel first of all.

MANNERISM

Pathos, because it is genuine self-expression, underlines the individual's characteristics without conscious effort. To be true, it must be unaffected and unwilled. A person who fools himself may have real pathos, but the person who merely wishes to fool others has none. He has mannerisms.

The neurotic person belongs in a special category. He certainly deviates from genuine self-expression. Affectations can easily become his pattern, but this happens unwilled because the emotions are uncontrolled. He does not want to play a part. He plays it because he accepts it as genuine expression.

Mannerism is the caricature of pathos. It is always willed to conceal something or to embellish oneself in the eyes of others, or to acquire something or conquer someone by fraudulent means. But first and most of all, mannerism always clamors for attention. It is vocal exhibitionism.

Mannerism can be easily diagnosed, because it is unphysiological. It uses a range that is not the true range of the speaker and a nasal resonance that is in no relation to the emotional content of the words. It plays on a register that is not normal and that did not grow but was made. It may permeate all phases of speech, respiration, phonation, articulation, and may involve every part of the vocal mechanism, including the resonator and all facial muscles participating in mimics. Since inhalation and exhalation can be modified at will, mannerism governs them easily.

It is hard to separate individual mannerisms from culturally grafted ones. Love-making today borrows words from the movies, whereas in former times the love-maker had to invent his personal speech melody. The influence of "canned" voices is so important that it is practically impossible not to be affected by these set vocal patterns. It follows that mannerism is never creative, never a new form for a new content. It is like speaking in superlatives. This is why it so painfully affects people with creative hearing, just as does the pathological voice. A typical example is the radio commentator who sells the international situation and his sponsor's toothpaste with equal enthusiasm.

Some "refined" mannerisms are the desperate gesture to escape one's group, just as the use of slang by those not yet familiar with the language indicates the wish to belong, or to seem to belong.

False paternalism, expressed through a fraudulent voice, hides lack of authority. Overcompensation is a contributing cause. But the stuffed shirt's harsh, brisk voice is not necessarily that of a neurotic. The starched shirt front merely bolsters a weakling. It is the vocal equivalent of the elevator shoe, the uniform which lends stature to someone who feels inadequate. One must keep in mind that the use of mannerisms is often a pre-stage to neurosis, since it has no lasting effect. Their use is an attempt to convey feelings that are not felt, convictions that are advertising copy, dignity that is a mirage. The insecurity will break through when the artificiality has outlived its functions. The cardboard house will collapse with the first drastic traumatic experience, and the poor actor will become a sad patient.

MELISM

Melism is the vocal means of expressing personal appeal.[48] It differs from mannerism in that it is always sincere, and it differs from pathos in that it is not necessarily unconscious. To be effective, however, it must possess finesse. It is the hairline brush touch in a painting, the minute variation on a main musical theme. It can consist of an imperceptible ritardando or acceleration, of a minuscule pause, a slight glide in pitch, or the tiniest inflection so small as to be immeasurable. Melism can make a simple statement a compliment or make it ironical. Here again one recognizes the clumsiness of our written symbols. Suspicion expressed by voice is the product of melism.

When the appeal ceases to be sincere, melism is transformed into mannerism. This transition is especially evident in the hysteric personality, where the variations between genuine expression and half-willed play-acting have become patterns. The diagnostician must train his ear to detect these indicative vocal variations and not depend on his instincts.

REGULARITY, UNIFORMITY, EXACTNESS

These vocal characteristics are not dimensions that are measurable and isolatable. Neither are they complex, unmeasurable factors like pathos or mannerism. They can be described fully although they pertain to a pattern of co-ordination. We use the term *"regularity"* to denote the repetition of one or more vocal qualities at regular intervals, or in recurring response to certain stimuli. For example, a speaker might use stereotyped habits, stick to particular vocal expressions, and even his interjections such as h-m-m-m-, harrumph, and a-a-a-h could be identical in pitch and duration. Less extreme instances may show merely a use of the same vowel length when varying emotional situations would call for different timing. One warning must be made: so-called nervous habits should not be confused with articulatory difficulties. Unless one is able to articulate flexibly, his speech cannot be termed regular or irregular. Once an individual has learned how to articulate, however, regularity and irregularity assume psychological significance.

Regularity, while not as all-inclusive as uniformity, makes a voice less adaptable and more predictable. One knows what is coming. Too much regularity may mean a low I. Q. It may imply the stereotyped behavior of the conventional—dullness, lack of imagination— or it may be the pedantic pattern of the inhibited, the retentive person who does not wish to disclose the warp from which his emotions are woven. Good manners can be a disguise to hide unbridled passion. Stereotyped, regular, conventional speaking may serve the same purpose.

Too little regularity, unexpected variations of small detail which surprise the speaker as well as the listener, portray the capricious individual who communicates all the shadings of his emotions, relevant and irrevelant, as well as the person whose urges outdistance his will power. It may mean lack of interest in others, exhibitionism, and poorly organized mental processes.

Irregularity gives color to speech as long as the variations stay within harmonious proportions. Here the law of esthetics applies. Vocal features or patterns that jar on the ears of average listeners are out of proportion, either absolutely or in the judgment of contemporary taste. In either case they indicate deviations from the norm. It has already been mentioned that patterns of speech acceptable fifty years ago can be deviations today, as demonstrated by recordings.

Uniformity: Uniformity shows itself not merely in the regular repetition of individual features or groups of features but in the entire process of phonation. There is an element of compulsive muscular rigidity that does not permit volitional alterations of movements. Regularity allows for variation; uniformity does not. In an extreme instance of uniformity, muscular tenseness would amount to complete physical stupor prohibiting any expansive movement, including respiratory expansion. In a less extreme instance, with speech still possible, tenseness could still restrict voice, articulation and respiration because of a contraction of the diaphragm and a retracted position of the abdominal muscles. General tenseness involves contraction of pharyngeal and neck muscles which should not be used in phonation, and the resulting strain is audible. For lower tones, vocal cords must be relaxed. This is the reason that uniformity characterized by tenseness cannot produce tones at the lower end of the scale.

The opposite of uniformity is variety. This does not mean freedom to let our vocal powers run wild under the impact of impulses and urges. When we are extremely tense, our will power is paralyzed. Muscles do not obey but remain fixed in spite of volition to move them. Variability predicates the orderly management of impulses and responses:

> O constancy! Be strong upon my side;
> Set a huge mountain 'tween my heart and tongue.
> *Julius Caesar, iv 6*

Extreme variability is as pathological as extreme uniformity, since it is a sign of the disorganization of willful control.

Uniformity in speech is always a pathological symptom. It characterizes the genuinely depressed voice even when the uniformity is present only to a limited degree. As mentioned before, King Edward VIII's farewell speech is a good example of depressed uniformity. The voice which has great variability within the limits of harmonic proportion, a way of speaking wherein no one feature dominates disproportionately, is the voice of the many-faceted, perceptive person. Some psychologists maintain that as a person matures, he becomes less flexible, less manifold in his potentialities; they say he becomes more unified, and in a sense more limited. Variability thus should be characteristic of the "eternally young," of whom one may choose to approve or disapprove. One may call these people immature, lacking real emotional stability, adventurers, influencable, opportunistic; or one may call them sensitive, compassionate, responsive, creative—depending on one's own point of view and sympathies. Being flexible, such people have a good measure of both plus and minus characteristics.

Exactness: Exactness entails greater respiratory pressure and better abdominal support, exact pitch without too much glissando, well co-ordinated resonance and careful articulation. All these elements can be measured by instruments and the resulting perfected oral movements can be seen by the naked eye. When exactness is exaggerated, it can also be distinguished by the ear.

There is a wide range in exactness. It extends from the excessive inexactitude of general paresis, which was formerly often diagnosed from this typical speech pattern, to the over-exactness of compulsion, with many in-between stages which are within normal limits. Exactness in speech is a willed effort and a result of training. Its absence or presence to any degree will shed light on psychological states and processes.

To examine the areas of interpretation of regularity, uniformity and exactness, one must keep in mind that regularity and uniformity relate to the flow of speech; exactness can be analyzed at any random moment, a snapshot apart from the rest. Because exactness is a result of training, it indicates rationality and power of concentration. An intelligent person, not emotionally unbalanced, will speak with a fair amount of exactness. A good teacher, concerned with being understood by his students, will, on the whole, speak exactly and so will a polite, considerate person. On the negative end of the scale, there is the exactness of the pedant, which can mean "This is it; this is the right way, the way I do it." This implies also a lack of perceptiveness and receptiveness as far as others are concerned. Or it may express less overcompensation and a rather anxious desire for not being misunderstood. A person speaking down to his audience will also endeavor to speak exactly.

The person who has inhibitions against spontaneous expression may also speak with exactitude, slowly and in a limited range. Depending on the degree of inhibition and the combination with other elements, this can indicate self control, repression, or a retentiveness—an unwillingness to give or to disclose oneself. The over-exactness which stems from a narcissistic oral gratification and the attendant pleasure of listening to one's own vocal play may, with luck, be sublimated into good artistic expression if it includes the gift of a superior voice. Good singers love to sing and love to hear themselves sing. A good speaker, however, must concern himself more with the content of his speech and the manipulation of his audience than with self-gratification. For this one needs more than a good voice and a good ear.

Lack of exactness does not mean naturalness per se. Many actors and radio artists today make the semantic mistake of using inexact speech for fear of appearing mannered; sometimes they do this to the extent of not being understood.

An impulsive person never speaks exactly, but if he is intelligent and not emotionally unbalanced the inexactness will not be too great or impede understanding. One may speak inexactly either because he does not wish to communicate or because he does not care whether he is understood. The withdrawn person, as well as the rude person, therefore, may be inexact in various degrees. When inexactness is temporary, it may show that emotional impulses have the upper hand of volitional control. It may show lack of co-ordination between impulse and rationality.

Inexact speech can be the direct expressional result of neurosis, or it can be due to an allergy caused by emotional conflict which impairs the functions of the vocal apparatus.

THE LISTENING PROCESS

To be confronted with the patient in the office does not allow for much more than the use of intuition. The voice analyst is distracted by the speakers' looks, gestures and his general behavior.

For an objective investigation a good tape recorder is preferable. In most cases the patient can know that a microphone is being used. The material for analysis should contain at least fifteen to twenty sentences. The easiest procedure is a dialogue situation. In reading aloud most people, especially women, raise the pitch of their voices. Therefore spontaneous speech is preferable. Occasionally the discrepancy between speaking spontaneously and reading aloud can be used for diagnostic purposes. The importance of divorcing the voice from the content of the words and the difficulty of doing so cannot be stressed enough. The recording must be played several times to the point where the content is absorbed and no longer interests the listener. This is no waste motion. Some vocal elements of meaningful speech as distinguished from singing are determined by content, and the repetition fixes this relationship firmly in the listener's mind. After the content ceases to impress, one is ready to observe the intuitive reactions to the voice. At first the voice as a whole plays on the analyst's feelings. This step somewhat resembles the method employed by listening studies in psychology departments, where the reaction to the voice by the student is of greater interest than the psychological features of the speaker. At first the heard voice may bring to mind anything, or nothing in particular. These first impressions will be set aside as soon as one can concentrate on the individual vocal features. They should not prejudice the ear. One is never able to recapture them after having, so to speak, dissected the living voice.

It is important to emphasize that this freedom from prejudice is not some personal endowment, nor is it a dexterity that is acquired with great discipline. It needs to be learned but it is simple enough to do so. The prejudice is usually based upon a dominant feature that reminds us of the voice of someone else. As soon as we perceive the relationship of this dominant to the other vocal elements, the similarity fades and usually disappears. Occasionally, instead of a single prominent feature, the coordination of the voice seems similar. The experience is something like seeing a stranger and being startled by his resemblance to a friend only to discover on second glance that none of his features show any likeness.

The record must be played over for each dimension, sometimes more than once. The dimension most easily isolated is that of speed. Does the person speak slowly or fast? How long are the pauses between words and between sentences? Next comes volume. Does the patient speak loudly or softly, is the general intensity changing? Does the patient often pause for a new breath? Which is the longer, inhalation, or exhalation? Can either or both be heard? Is either forced?

Is the range wide or limited? Does the voice break or is it even? Does the speaker use many dynamic accents? Does he emphasize much or little? Is accentuation in accord with meaning? Does the speaker lower the pitch at the end of sentences or does he raise his voice even when he does not ask a question?

Some of the melodic and rhythmic aspects are more difficult to follow than these simpler elements but after a certain number of repetitions, they to become disentangled. One should write down his observations while examining the voice, concentrating entirely on factual observation and description, and leave interpretation to the last when all notes are completed.

After describing as exhaustively as possible the individual features of the voice, one starts looking into their relationships. First of all, one notes whether there is a dominant attribute and if so, what it is. For example, a voice might immediately impress by its tempo, not only because this is the easiest dimension to perceive but because the person speaks rapidly. Then one listens for the second dominant, a feature that does not command attention so insistently but is nevertheless noticeable. It may be clarity in accentuation or the lack of it. One notes the important relationship of the two dominants. Many vocal elements are psychologically ambivalent and their directional value is disclosed in relation to other elements. For example, a fast speaking voice with marked dynamic accents indicates positive traits: forcefulness, enthusiasm, quick perception. Which element depends on the other is an additional feature. A fast speaking voice conspicuously lacking accents or indistinct or wrongly accented suggests negative traits, such as superficiality, stupidity, or even feeble-mindedness.

Before attempting any interpretation, one observes the relationship of all dimensions of the voice and the important subpatterns of pathos, melism, and mannerism, exactness or inexactness in phonation and articulation, and regularity and uniformity, or their opposites in the flow. It is only then that one begins to put the puzzle together on the interpretive level of personality expression and the specific features of the neurotic voice.

A few warnings are in order here. At this stage one may be tempted to correct the first impressions jotted down under the influence of intuition. This one should never do. First of all, whether or not they are confirmed by the findings, one should keep documentary evidence of first reactions. The more they are studied, the more one compares them with the objectively acquired results and with subsequent first reactions tempered by greater experience, the more one learns about personal equation—the personal bias for which one must make allowances. Secondly, because of the newness and relative crudeness of this method of analysis or because of lack of skill, it might well happen that intuition was truer than labored analysis. One is just as liable to make an error in observation as in intuitive understanding. Intuition is merely a shortcut judgment based on previous experience. Discrepancies between first impressions and findings will prompt us to repeat our observations until the nature of the error is detected.

One of the main obstacles confronting a beginner when he listens to a voice is very much a part of this personal bias. In intuition one leaves the mental doors open to free association and one cannot prevent like or dislike from forcing itself into consciousness. When one listens to a heart murmur one does not experience likes and dislikes. One merely notes what one hears and interprets it in the light of previous diagnostic experience. The interfering emotional responses can be removed by finding their causes.

In interpreting individual features and patterns of coordination the beginner is often greatly handicapped by his preoccupation with dissection, sometimes euphemistically called "fact finding," coupled with a complete inability to put the pieces together again. This attitude, as well as the urge to "score" mathematically without giving allowance to individual, racial, environmental, and cultural implications, has often blocked the road to vocal analysis for the psychologist.

CHAPTER V

Areas of Interpretation in the Neurotic Personality

NEUROSIS IS MANY THINGS to many people. There is lack of agreement not only among sufferers and laymen but among psychiatrists as well. Obviously the depth of this theoretical jungle cannot be explored here. For working purposes, however, a few guiding principles should be laid down.

Fenichel[49] describes neurotic symptoms as strange and unintelligible to the patient, whether they be involuntary movement, changes in bodily functions and various sensations, overwhelming and unjustified moods, or "queer" impulses or thoughts. Something from an unknown source breaks in upon his personality from outside the realm of his conscious will. When symptoms overtake the whole personality, character-neurosis originates. In all these conditions, the crux is the insufficiency of the normal control apparatus. The patient's neurosis is an unsuccessful attempt to solve a problem in the present by means of a behavior pattern that failed to solve it in the past.

Neurotic symptoms, that is, failure of control, develop from the basic tendency of all living organisms to achieve control over their internal and external environment. While all processes of living involve a cumulative tension, release from tension reestablishes homeostasis. When the release fails to come or fails to bring expected readjustment, the individual will try to find substitute avenues. The neurotic individual whose release has been frustrated by external or internal obstacles will find emotionally costly and involved substitutes, while the non-neurotic will adapt in a more economical manner. To understand the mechanics of neurosis, especially in vocal expression, one must bear in mind that the basic aspect of human relations between individuals, between individuals and

81

groups, and between groups is the opportunity for the full expression of each relationship.

Communication is a basic aspect of social living. The organ used in communication unavoidably registers the frustrations and byways of neurotic adaptation as against normal reactions. Frustration originates through the not understood message. There is no doubt that the whole vocal apparatus is affected by these frustrated attempts and that the attempt to overcome the frustration puts new burdens on the voice. Ruesch[50] calls neurosis "difficulties in the area of transmission of messages to others."

Not only do all neuroses have vocal symptoms of some kind, whether or not the patient or physician notices them, but certain failures of control will directly affect the channel of communication. Here again a distinction must be made between neuroses which affect behavior in a way involving misuse or abuse of the vocal apparatus and neuroses where control of the vocal mechanism itself fails. This distinction is important because the vocal muscles are volitionally controlled. The first type of disorder may take the form of a bad habit, like those developed after some acute illness; while the second has a mechanical cause and resembles more closely other psychosomatic diseases.

Normal emotional reactions can be mistaken for neuroses. "Nervousness" is an acute deviation from the usual emotional tonus. Everyone is nervous at times without necessarily being neurotic. Expectation of an oppressive situation, such as an examination, or of a painful event, such as childbirth or surgery, pushes the individual out of homeostasis. Vocally the nervous person will step out of his normal pattern and his reactions will vary according to the nature of the stimulus. The neurotic, on the other hand, will react with a set pattern to certain emotional situations and to situations that are in some way associated with them even when the connection is remote. In advanced cases the "normal" vocal pattern may be completely eliminated and the set neurotic co-ordination may govern all reactions. For example, a normal person may speak with a complaining inflection if annoyed, but a neurotic may use this inflection constantly, having, as it were, forgotten how to speak in an uncomplaining manner.

The non-neurotic voice will fit the occasion, whereas the neurotic voice will show the pattern, independent of situations. This voice, pathological in itself, will eventually produce audible and sometimes visible symptoms. The patient will present typical complaints of hoarseness, vocal fatigue, pain, hyper- or hyposecretion, paresthesia, cough; in short, the whole complex of complaints typical of myasthenia or phonasthenia. In spite of all these inconveniences he continues using the "wrong voice," which gives us reason to believe that something stronger than pain and discomfort *forces* him to maintain this insufficient use of vocal cords. Often the careful observer has the impression that the patient is expressing through body language: "I would rather be hoarse than communicate."

Neurosis in itself is voice-bound. One can safely say that the majority of neuroses has an almost characteristic vocal expression. On the other hand, from the voice can be gained an insight into the nature of the expressed neurosis.

Vocal expression, however, is time-bound. The normal way our great-grandmothers spoke might be considered highly neurotic today. Had they spoken in their time with the voices of the present generation, they would have been considered, to say the least, peculiar. These changing vocal fashions are easily understood by comparing the vocal expression of the movies during the last twenty years. The experience of voice through the listener needs to become the subject of scientific observation. Instead of using purely intuitive methods, the voice must be analyzed according to objective principles.

It is impossible even to sketch areas of the neurotic voice without drawing a map which shows the outlines of normal personality. Personality is the living, breathing entity in all its dynamics: development, degeneration, creativeness and destructiveness. It is never still, never in equilibrium. That is an individual. Cicero said, "Mens cuiusque est quisque." The mind of each man is the man himself. This is not too broad a definition to be scientifically useful and it avoids static implications.

The word character is related to the Greek word for an etching instrument. Originally it was used for single traits; today however, "characteristics" means the sum of the traits that make up personality. One therefore may interpret character as being the aggregate of an individual's traits at any given moment. It is, as it were, a short-exposure portrait of a personality. A so-called normal personality is never at rest except when it ceases to exist. There is no fixation in the sense of standing still, no regression in the sense of return, no maturity in the sense of final solution. The developmental limits are flexible and unknown as yet, but the fact of motion, flux, dynamics is incontestable. In this sense, too, voice is a highly appropriate medium to mirror the mental physiognomy of the individual because its essence is movement and all its qualities and attributes are dynamic.

Personality research, quite apart from research into vocal expression, is still in its infancy. Analytical methods vary from depth analysis, an historical reconstruction of the inner structure of the individual, to behaviorism, which concerns itself more with manifestations than with motivations. Because of present day preoccupation with quantifications, batteries of tests are constructed to measure this and that, occasionally on an astonishingly childish level. There are both the mathematic method, expressing complex phenomena by adding scores of less than ten; and the psychological method which takes as "objective" norms the knowledge and value judgments of a specific culture or a restricted geographic or economic group. These methods certainly cannot be applied in describing and analyzing vocal features and they cannot be used for tests of normal or neurotic personality.

Vocal expression in neurosis has to be considered from the viewpoint of heredity and environment. Unfortunately the most heated scientific debates center around this very question. Another controversial subject is the role of constitution and/or training in the formation of personality, and consequently its expression. Menninger[51] assumes that "functional propensities are usually acquired rather than inherited." If we appraise voice in this context, we must ask: Is a particular voice produced by "functional propensities" or is it the product of structurally determined organs? Or is it a mixture, and if so, of how much is each composed? There is no doubt that the human voice with its particular expressiveness, quality and attributes is as much a mixture of constitutional (inherited and accidental) factors and of environmental influences as is the personality itself. Menninger tries to define environmental factors as those which as yet cannot be controlled. With regard to voice, range (tenor, baritone, basso) would be hereditary, whereas the *use* of range, or intensity, for instance, is subject to environmental and cultural influences.

Not much is known about the prenatal development of the endocrine system. And yet this shapes and regulates much of our morphology and our functioning. The "mosaic of androgyny," the composite of masculine and feminine characteristics in a grown individual, is set, at least in its structural potential, before birth and so is our growth potential. By the time the infant is born he is stamped indelibly with the morphological and energy potentials which, within limits, will determine his personal identity throughout life. This androgynic mixture and proportion exists audibly in the normal voice. However, the neurotic voice often reveals the constituents in a more conspicuous way. This feature actually started a new era in vocal-morphological research. In 1921 Dalma[52] found higher voices in schizophrenics than in other psychopaths. The author, in rechecking these·findings, came to different conclusions. The increased use of isolated registers is characteristic of schizophrenics (see Conclusion).

Beginning with this the author described vocal attitudes of the schizoid type. Even if Kretschmer's and Sheldon's theories are built too much from a static point of view, one cannot help recognizing that the congenital body characteristics often fall into certain well definable types. In psychopathology I have tried with fair success to trace these schizoid and pyknic types among schizophrenics and manic-depressives. It will be demonstrated later that vocal (dynamic) features show these characteristics much more than any of the morphological features. The schools of thought that reduce human behavior and motivation to endocrine or biochemical functions are not too far advanced over the morphologists. They give a somewhat broader scope to internal processes, as differentiated from external manifestations. Fundamentally, however, they are closely related to the mechanistic approach which was popular a century or so ago, and which reduced human behavior to a response to outward stimulation. These newer theories merely changed "outward" to "inward" stimulation.

The neurotic voice contains genetic, congential and constitutional determinants, as contrasted to environmental ones. So does the non-neurotic voice. These determinants can be more easily identified in the neurotic than in the normal voice. Since hyper- and hypofunction often produce a caricature of the original vocal procedure, it is easier to hear the potential range in excited patients. In the balanced attitudes, as mentioned earlier, we hear the lowest third only. Under excitement the higher range will break, the registers will split, the character of the registers will be audible. In this instance we hear genetic features not influenced by an intrauterine environment. Range can almost be determined by the laws of heredity (see Chapter III).

During puberty these registers are subject to gonadothropic influence in their quantity and in their quality. This is the time when the relative mixture of secondary sex characteristics is shaped and the result shows in the androgyny of the individual's voice. In singers the proportions are increased. Lyric voices in men reveal more femaleness; dramatic voices in women reveal more maleness. The lyric voices have increased head register; the dramatic ones increased chest register. The same rules hold in the proportions of the speaking voice. This femaleness in men becomes evident under neurotic conditions when the head register is used in an isolated way. It comes out in its most exaggerated form in schizophrenics.

The neurotic conditions expressed through persistent falsetto voice reveal almost in caricature the identical changes which take place in normal puberty. In puberty they are perhaps less audible. Under the influence of changing sex glands and as a pituitary coordinate, the voice often breaks over a long period of time. In non-neurotic conditions this phase usually has less marked audible phenomena.

Climacteric Voice: In males the climacteric voice is the voice that loses volume and strength. The range becomes narrower and often higher. Occasionally there is complete divergence of registers and tremolo. Female subfunctions of the sex glands can become audible in *menarche*. This comes from lowering the voice, from engorged nasal turbinates, sneezing, occasional rhinorrhea. These are organic symptoms which under neurotic conditions become much more pronounced, as do subfunctions in the male.

Changes in the thyroid gland often occur under emotional influences. These changes nearly always cause some vocal symptoms. This is especially true in professional speakers and singers who suffer from varying hyper- and hypofunctions of the thyroid. They complain often about symptoms which contain practically the whole symptomatology of phonasthenia: hoarseness, vocal fatigue, pressure symptoms on neck and throat, dryness and inability to project the voice. All these occur under trying emotional situations.

Twenty years ago anxiety was regarded as a symptom of hyperthyroidism. Today it is believed that the reverse may be just as true. Moreover, anxiety may be a symptom of many other conditions in addition to hyperthyroidism, among them hypothyroidism. Since the endocrine glands are coordinated in such a complex manner, few if any psychological symptoms can be attributed to the function of any single gland.

Speculation about the functional relationship between voice and bodily structure has been advanced since antiquity. But the history of morphology and phenomenology credits Giovanbattista della Porta,[53] a Neopolitan physician who lived from 1545 to 1615, with the first systematic attempt to analyze the voice. He searched for analogies between animals and human beings. He compared every human type to some animal whose physiognomy bore a likeness to the human and he tried to find a resemblance in their respective voices. More important, Porta took Galen's morphological types and fitted them with appropriate voices. His observations in this regard were acute. For example, he found that Galen's hot mixture, the man who had a rough, hot skin, a lean body, ruddy complexion, coarse, black, curly hair and prominent veins, breathed audibly and spoke in a loud voice. The cool mixture, on the other hand, which displayed a fatless, slowly developing body, cool skin, pale sallow complexion and scant hair of fine texture, breathed softly and slowly and spoke with a thin, sharp voice. Porta also described intermediate mixtures and characterized these vocally.

The study of voice as an expression of personality, constitutional and psychological, has been continued sporadically since Porta. However, the problem has been treated as a step-child by modern psychology. Only in pathology has some attention been paid to it, because the vocal symptoms of certain nervous and mental afflictions were too obvious to be passed over.

Before presenting illustrative material of the most important vocal features of neurosis and psychosis, some drives and traits will be presented as areas of interpretation.

The drive for autonomy, whether successful or unsuccessful, can be interpreted either as a tendency to act as one pleases or as the building of a successful ego. Pathos, the threshold of ego expression, has been discussed previously. It reflects rather conclusively the direction as well as the intensity of the drive for autonomy. It will vary with developmental stages of the individual. Obviously pathos will be different in early childhood when the child first discovers he is a distinct entity. It will differ in adolescence when he must choose courses to follow for his whole future, one direction or another. It will differ again in so-called maturity when he must resist the impact of his surroundings in order to maintain the integrity of his ego with success.

Before the child can become a separate entity, he must establish communication. The child goes through a period of identification, imitation, borrowing, and acceptance before he can begin to form his own ego. The corresponding vocal process was described in Chapter II. What was described, however, was fundamentally more the adaptability of the voice as such to surrounding early influences. Ego building is a painful process, from being weened from mother's breast to the discovery of the existence of competition for mother's attention, both people and objects. It is hard to face nursery school contemporaries who have different rhythms and identities. All these traumatic experiences leave scars which are audible in the neurotic voice.

Adaptability is an important factor for survival. The adaptable child will identify himself easily with groups and individuals. His voice will show distinct stereotypes well into adolescence. But if ego formation is never achieved or is postponed, one faces the appalling adult who hides behind the skirts of his family, his social club, his party, his nationality or race. He claims superiority not by virtue of achievement but by "belonging." Vocally these people retain and remain stereotypes all their lives. They will tell a joke with exactly the same inflection as the speaker at the annual dinner, and their language will be studded with "loaded" concepts.

Successful ego formation is based on successful identification. In adolescence, when the pendulum is still in full swing between mother and a non-incestuous object of desire, registers express the direction and intensity of the drive for autonomy.

Vocally the marks of the self-assured, the successful ego are a harmonious, balanced co-ordination and a relaxed operating diaphragm. Dry, tense vocal cords, excessive pathos, overemphasis are signs of the struggle of the individual who hits back at an environment rather than attempting to overcome and change it.

The drive for achievement shows vocal variations which correspond to different motivations. Achievement may be sought because of real interest or showmanship, and because it gives pleasure, directly or indirectly. Finally, it may be a form of ego building, a pathos of will that compels the individual to challenge his surroundings. The voice of defeat in this drive will lack the specific expression which characterizes the voice of successful achievement. The missing pathos of will can be heard through slower speed, unclear articulation, inexactness, lesser variation in the dynamics of volume and intensity, and lesser rhythmic qualities. The last syllable in a declarative sentence will often fail to fall downward in direction; chest register will not be predominant.

Narcissistic drive for achievement can be a simple conversion of primitive sexual exhibitionism. In singers it takes the form of producing single tones or groups of tones that please, without necessarily having an interest in the musical or artistic qualities of the composition. These singers take pride in the beauty or volume or length of the tone they can produce. They will have tremendous appeal for the majority of the audience which will participate in the exhibitionistic act with the relish of peeping Toms. This type of singer will center his interest on how long he can hold high C. He will sing it with the expression of achievement. He will hold it up, a perfect example of voice symbolizing the sex organ which includes the semantic meaning that "high" means "high."

Lack of social adjustment is shown in the attempt to conform to the speaking habits of the group. Here the role of mannerism enters, mannerism resembling the true article, although a sensitive and auditively trained ear will recognize it as a sham. Social maladjustment does not express itself uniformly because the voice will show the correlation to the basic reasons for the maladjustment. Both an indifferent and an oversensitive person may not be adjusted to their surroundings, but their vocal portraits will differ.

Some commonplace, generally recognized emotional states show their vocal expressions more clearly.

The complainer feels sorry for himself. According to his vertical state of mind, he is far down—in a depression. Vocally he will express this in the range he uses. He will speak deep down but he fights his depression. Were he not to do this, he would not complain. The attempt to climb up again measures the degree of his constriction. The free energy used to climb is manifest in a continuity of upward tendencies in his melody. The usual vocal pattern of complaining is a constantly up and down gliding pitch.

There is no complaining without accusation. In German the semantics of the related verbs is most revealing: *klagen, beklagen, anklagen.* The first means complaining in general, the second complaining specifically about something or someone (also mourning), the third means accusing. The English word stems from the *Latin plangere:* to beat, to strike one's breast. The masochistic element is in the word but all masochism has its compensating fraction of sadism. Complaining depresses the listener. It wants to elicit sympathy, companionship in suffering, and this means inflicting this suffering on others while asking for succor. The vocal dynamics of complaining bear witness to this ambivalence. Like self-accusation

"Mea culpa, mea culpa, mea maxima culpa," complaint beats on the breast of the complainer with its insistent rhythm and at the same time it wants to beat on the ear and conscience of the listener. It combines the request for help and accusation.

The quarrelsome. Complaining is a release from a state of mind. The complainer needs a shoulder to cry on. However, the owner of the shoulder need not necessarily be directly involved in the situation. But quarreling is possible only with a partner and it is the existence of this partner which acts as the provocation. It is obvious that in quarreling, aggressive vocal features are prominent. Dynamics are stressed. The melody is expressive of the following feelings: (1) I am innocent. (2) I am hurt. (3) I know how to fight. (4) I stand on my rights. (5) Why do you hurt me? (6) This is the last time.

Vocally these implications sound as follows: (1) Self-assertion which guides the melody downward. (2) Pain starts with a glottal stroke, loudly; then it glides into a lower pitch with decreased intensity. (3) Is an exhibition of alleged strength with emphatic dynamic accents. (4) Implies righteous indignation in a chest tone of conviction; *i.e.,* chesty register mixture. (5) Is a question which mixes into the medley a rising inflection. (6) Maintains, throughout, the strength of dynamic accents. The grasping features of ego-insistence are heard in the sustained dynamic accents.

These are stereotypes of vocal expression, persistent factors in communication, indications of character traits which often play a part in neurotic expression. Before entering typical vocal patterns of neurosis we will sum up some physiognomical characteristics of the voice as such. This can be done in a tentative, empirical arrangement of the most obvious vocal patterns as encountered in clinical experience, but not in rigid classification. The following categories are not mutually exclusive.

(1) *Conscious and unconscious voices.* There may exist an inner censor which controls expression consciously. The voice may then be either conventionalized or noticeably controlled by will; or it may be self-conscious, embarrassed. Or it may be mannered.

The voice that is not consciously guided may also be conventionalized as a result of environmental influence and adaptability. It may be objectivized or reactive, or it may have much or little pathos, depending on other traits of the speaker.

(2) *Subjective or objective voices.* A subjective voice discloses directly a great deal about the speaker. Objective voices are used primarily for the communication of content and secondarily as a shield behind which the ego hides.

(3) *Active and reactive voices.* Active voices are manipulative. They have appeal and they create in the listener an intended reaction. Reactive voices on the other hand, while they may have appeal, are primarily conditioned by situations rather than by the intention of the speaker.

CASE HISTORIES

Case 1.

Mrs. A. L., aged 39 years, was a woman of agreeable appearance, intelligent, educated, in comfortable circumstances. She did not seem to present any special problems. Her complaint was hoarseness, formerly diagnosed as due to "weakness of the vocal cords." Most of the time she talked or pronounced on inspiratory voice. Her voice constantly wavered. She stopped for deep inhalation after every three or four syllables. The only significant physical finding was incomplete closure of the vocal cords.

There was a good relationship with her quiet, rather unexceptional husband. She had no children of her own but brought up a niece, then 14 years old.

This idyllic picture was disturbed on the peripheries. Her aggressive, domineering mother lived in the same apartment house, constantly attempting to interfere with the couple's life. The patient's sister, mother of the niece, was a thrice-divorced alcoholic, completely uncontrolled and uncontrollable, who lived in the same community and "associated with all kinds of undesirable elements." Mrs. L. was a warm, outgoing, frank individual. Some of her voice difficulty started in childhood when she was condemned to silence by a mother who "knew everything better and had all the answers." Mrs. L.'s effort to keep her niece, the center of her life, ignorant of her alcoholic mother's condition and activities increased her repressions and led to the development of a full-fledged neurosis. Expressional therapy was successful. The patient recognized the source of her trouble and understood well the relation between keeping a secret and talking in inspiratory voice. Her voice became stronger, less wavering, and the intake of breath less frequent. Since it was impossible to change the outside circumstances decisively, no complete cure could be expected at the time.

Case 2.

Mrs. C. T., aged 29 years, was treated for "chronic laryngitis" before being referred. Examination showed her larynx to be normal, with very slightly irritated vocal cords which, however, during phonation came to an almost spastic closure. She spoke in a pressed, almost voiceless manner while inhaling air. She was therefore hardly intelligible. She first experienced extreme hoarseness in the midst of an embarrassing courtroom scene. This was soon followed by inability to talk normally without undue strain.

Her dramatics history was revealed voluntarily in the course of treatment. At the age of 18 she married a man much older than herself, against her parents' wishes. The marriage could take place only after complicated divorce proceedings from the man's first wife. Hardly back from their honeymoon, the husband started to drink heavily and to behave in a generally irresponsible manner. She tried to conceal the situation from her parents through fear of their saying "We told you so." After ten years the situation became intolerable. She finally sought divorce but still could not bring herself to admit to her parents that she had lost the battle. She kept her divorce and her troubles a secret from the family. Here, as in Case 1, the patient's natural tendencies were not retentive. She did not like to have secrets. She was forced by circumstances to dam up practically unendurable pressure. The supreme effort she made not to talk about her troubles engulfed the whole of the voice. The prolonged tension was transferred to the vocal cords and she spoke inward instead of outward. Within six weeks after treatment was begun her voice was greatly improved by exercises for expiratory phonation. But these mechanical aids would have been of little use had not talking out her troubles and understanding the mechanism brought about catharsis and understanding.

Case 3.

Mrs. F. R., aged 58 years, came to the Clinic because of weakness of voice and inability to carry on any long conversation. Although her voice had not been strong for many years, she had felt actually handicapped by it for about two years. The vocal cords appeared normal. Phonation occurred under almost spastic approximation. Vocal production was made partly during inspiration, partly with symptoms of wavering. No other visible pathology could be found. For external reasons a truly expressive treatment could not be arranged in the ENT Clinic. The patient was referred to psychiatry where, after considerable hesitation on her part, the following history was explored: The patient's son was in the Army and was engaged to a girl whom the patient liked very much. This son had been born out of wedlock. The woman's conscience began to bother her. Did she need to reveal to her future daughter-in-law the secret of her life? When the son came back from Korea, the situation became almost intolerable and her formerly weak voice began the symptoms which could and still can be heard: it shifted from wavering but expiratory to an almost completely inspiratory function.

The psychiatrist decided that she did not have to tell her daughter-in-law about this secret, but the assurance did not help. She still reveals the same syndrome.

This case history shows the real relation between psychodynamics and vocal dynamics. Since the woman was not relieved from the pressure of her secret, she certainly carried on with her former vocal dynamics. It remains to be seen whether her voice will be helped if eventually her daughter-in-law becomes a confidant of this dark spot in her life.

Case 4.

Judge C. B., a very impressive appearing man, aged 52 years, was referred because his chronic laryngitis did not disappear under the usual therapeutic procedures. Hoarseness, vocal fatigue, feeling of strain when talking were the main symptoms. The vocal cords looked irritated, some-what red and slightly swollen. The chin was pressed towards the sternum during speech, which caused longitudinal compression of the trachea. This interfered with efficient respiration. There was also insufficient coordination between the abdominal and thoracic movements and this gave a groaning sound to his breathing. His range was extremely low, the register function was isolated chest. One easily perceived when talk-ing to the patient that he was not only a judge but he was also the law. His authority was emphatic and uncompromising. He did not come to find out what ailed him. So far as he was concerned, he suffered from laryngitis and he did not care to discuss underlying causes with the doctor. Overcompensation was so blatant that it made one guess the source. The patient did not volunteer information on the origin of his vocal difficulties. It was only through polite but firm insistence that he was finally moved to trace the history of his vocal, and implicitly his psychological, problem.

The judge's father was a domineering personality who held an important public position and demanded success from every member of his family. After his father's death, the mother took over the reins, although she was in her late 70's when the patient was under treatment. From her son's characterization, she was undoubtedly an overwhelming woman, to say the least. The patient kept away from her as much as he could. He provided her with all the comforts but often found himself too busy to visit her. Being intent on proving to the world that he had inherited his father's crown, he secretly feared that he could not sustain the pretense with his mother.

By representing the law, the patient made out of himself a super father image which he expressed by increased chest register and by lowering the range beyond sound into a noise quality. Therapy consisted of teaching the use of the natural range of voice, which was considerably higher. The hardest obstacle to overcome was the freak use of the glottal stroke. With exercises for soft attack, this too was corrected. It should be added that during the course of treatment the patient released his defensive attitude. He learned to speak freely about his personal problems and within the last two years he has found it easy to use his natural range and is never hoarse.

Case 5.

Mr. G. H., aged 52 years, business man, was referred after having been hoarse for 8 years. Speaking was so difficult for him that he could hardly attend to his daily duties, avoided social contacts outside business hours, was treated for chronic laryngitis. Examination revealed thickened, reddish vocal cords. The right false cord was somewhat protruding. Glottis closure was pressed. The voice was very low and loud without modification. Chest register and chest resonance were predominant. The range was quite limited. Dynamic accents were hardly used.

The history revealed repeated attacks of serious depressions in the past, although none had been experienced within the last twelve years.

The depressed individual does not want to expose a broad surface to the unfriendly world. He shrinks. His gestures and movements become inhibited and his vocal range narrows. Continued depression without

manic intervals freezes the behavior pattern into an increasingly rigid
mode. The voice becomes inelastic. The melody with continuously falling
rhythm and falling intervals becomes so restricted that it borders on
monotony. The depressed vocal pattern often creates functional disorders. In the case of this patient the vocal cords became overstretched
from the constant effort to speak in the deepest range. Since there is
little or no dynamics in the depressed vocal coordination, sounds become
equally loud in order to be understood. This imposed a further strain
on the patient's vocal mechanisms. Again, the trachea was depressed in
a longitudinal direction. This whole inefficient coordination was so rigidly
set that the only release from vocal strain was complete silence. In spite
of absence of melancholic spells for so many years, and in spite of a
satisfactory adjustment to life and work, the vocal pattern of his former
maladjustment persisted through automatization and habit formation. His
intelligence helped him to understand that his vocal symptoms were scars
from an otherwise successful battle and not needed any more; or as he
himself expressed it, "You mean one wears a dark suit to a funeral but
not to a wedding." Complete cure of this voice condition was reached
after two months of treatment, consisting of explanation, reassurance and
regular exercises in raising pitch and range.

Case 6.

Miss V. D., aged 62, entered the clinic completely aphonic. She
brought with her a complete previous history, as if she understood that
the general circumstances were important. Her left arm was in a sling.
She was an unmarried former singer and later became a singing teacher.
However, because of frequent vocal disturbances she had given up the
singing career and became a piano teacher. She had always lived with
her ailing mother and was her sole support. Her present aphonia had
started two years before when her mother, in attempting unaided to get
out of bed, broke her hip. The patient had to give up her voice students
and concentrated on teaching piano. But this too had become increasingly
difficult, as her mother needed more and more attention. Now she herself
had broken an arm.

Examination showed no sign of organic disorder. The only physical
finding was incomplete closure of the glottis during attempted phonation.
Examination of the vocal cords at once became successful therapy, at
least as far as vocal function was concerned. As is so often true in these
cases, the readiness to be cured is obvious. During laryngoscopy, with

tongue stretched out and while a very high-pitched vowel EE is pronounced, the patient represses any idea of communication. He does not connect this procedure with voice production and therefore completely loses his inhibitions. Consequently a rather clear tone often originates, as in this case. Then all that needs to be done is to change vowels: EE to A to O to OO; meanwhile gently releasing the tongue, which at first is kept out. Next, slowly, while constantly repeating the vowels, a long tone should be produced, followed by meaningless syllables, still avoiding any similarity to communication. If then the patient eventually produces three long syllables (I — go — out), then only can one tell him, "This was already a whole sentence." Should the patient lose his voice again during this first treatment, he has only to phonate with stretched out tongue while the therapist continues encouraging him with no excess emotion, but using rather a casual friendliness. The patient must take for granted that he has regained his voice. This will open the door to successful psychotherapy, as transference is more easily obtained if the therapist presents the patient with an accomplished fact and not a theory.

In the case of Miss V. D. a more profound therapy was certainly necessary since her relapsing voice trouble belonged to the previous history and was of long standing. Noting her distress at not being able to reach a higher singing range, it was explained to her that narrowing range was a common occurrence after menopause but that as compensation her lower range would probably be better and wider than before. She was also reassured that she could teach voice without forcefully transgressing her remaining range. This reassurance, together with her completely recovered speaking voice, paved the way for excellent contact, so that the true psychodynamics behind her symptoms could be explained. Aphonia is silence and silence is the symbol of death. The patient during her long years of servitude to a demanding invalid must have wished subconsciously many a time that her mother were dead. Then she punished herself for this wish, unconsciously too, in her most vulnerable spot, her voice. When her mother's latest accident occurred, which made life almost intolerable, the death wishes came back, probably in an innocent form. But the patient became engulfed in guilt and remorse. She now lost her voice completely. "Death" for "death-wish" expiated her sin. She broke her arm, as if to say, "Now I too am an invalid." Or even "Now I too am an invalid and thus cannot help you."

It was explained to her that these wishes were entirely natural, considering her troubled existence, because in reality her so-called death wishes had not gone further than wishing that her mother would be relieved from suffering. Nothing, however, helped as quickly as the fact that the patient learned to use her singing voice again, at least to the extent that she could resume her teaching profession. It was the only practicable means to sustain her recovery from total aphonia.

Case 7.

Mr. B. C. L. complained of frequent attacks of hoarseness and he feared that these might herald the end of his career. A slender, somewhat asthenic looking man, aged 50 years, married, with no children, he was a professional vaudeville performer, billed as the "only great singer with complete baritone and soprano voice."

Previous history revealed petit mal attacks since adolescence. His physique was unquestionably male, masculine pattern of pubic hair, face somewhat effeminate, body medium-sized with signs of undernourishment.

This patient had had a thorough vocal education and had studied with several well known teachers. His range was duofold. He had good training and a falsetto range which reached from f' sharp to a''. With some pressure he could sing from d' sharp to b''. He sounded like a somewhat sentimental lyric soprano and had sufficient vocal strength when it was needed.

His baritone, also lyric in character, ranged from E to f' and had a higher artistic quality than his soprano, although it was less trained. The remarkable physiological fact was that there was no bridge between these two voices. Had he been able to unify them and sing through both in gradual transition, he would have had a truly astonishing range and volume. Contrary to his soprano, which was in reality pure falsetto function using head register exclusively, the baritone function was well performed with well mixed registers. His speaking voice was too high in relation to his singing range but it was not a persistent falsetto voice.

This patient did not separate his registers spontaneously because of neurotic loss of control. On the contrary, the separation was carefully and artistically controlled. Yet there was an element which defied volition, the fact that he could not unify his two ranges. He could not produce any tones about f' with mixed register function.

It seems to be characteristic of the schizoid type to have in inclination to separate registers; for instance, to use head register for communication. Mr. B. C. L.'s personality presented at least some indications in this direction. He was a soft-spoken, rather pompous, insignificant looking man, friendly and somewhat obsequious in his manner. He emphatically denied any homosexual tendencies, claiming that his friendships with men were "ordinary." He married happily, too late to have children. He was an ardent cultist and believed in "ignoring hunger, disease and sadness in life." This was the reason why it was difficult to get information about his previous medical history. His seizures "did not bother him." He was unhappy because he was considered a freak, because he was unable to do more than impersonate. In these impersonations he first appeared dressed as a woman to sing soprano and then as a man to sing baritone. He professed serious artistic ambitions and was disturbed by his hoarseness. He wanted to know whether he should concentrate on his baritone.

The tendency to sing in male and female voice is decidedly a schizoid fact. It is reminiscent of the archaic tendency to unify the sexes—hermaphroditic ideals from the cradle of mankind. His tragedy was that he was born in the wrong century. Two hundred years ago falsettists were higly paid and honored artists in the most famous church choirs.

As mentioned before, he was full of mannerisms, thanking too much for anything and everything, using the most complicated sentence construction with loaded words, somewhat preaching. The diagnosis "epilepsy" could not be substantiated. He might have been a schizoid neurotic who demonstrated the voice of the schizoid under a magnifying glass. Cure was impossible for his voice. Endocrine changes often prevent vocal cords from maintaining an "artistic" range in the fifth decade of life. In this exceptional case of isolated use of two registers, the falsetto function could not be used any more for artistic purposes, and the baritone voice, with some added lower tones, became the only usable range. What occurred here can be observed frequently; the "male climacterium" deprives a singer of his highest tones but adds some tones in the lower range.

Case 8.

Mr. M. N., foreman of a lumber yard, complained of hoarseness which often increased so much that choking sensations were felt in and around the throat. These symptoms appeared whenever he got nervous. Since this patient had great responsibilities in the lumber yard, he was constantly worried. The crew which worked with lumber in the country was a constant insurance risk and he was responsible to the insurance company that every safety precaution be taken. He slept badly, thinking constantly of these security risks, and this followed him in nightmares from which he awoke aphonic, with choking sensations.

The previous history revealed that he grew up with eleven siblings on a small ranch in New Mexico almost two hundred miles from the next town. When he was eight years old, all the children had "croup" (possibly diphtheria), and ten children died. He and one brother survived. There was no medical help available. He saw them all die. Since then fear has meant choking to him, and the exaggerated anxiety which now penetrates his work has caused a non-ceasing pattern of hyperfunctions in his larynx. The situation was thoroughly explained to him. However, he had to leave before marked improvement could be observed.

Case 9.

Mr. J. R., aged 23, was referred by his fiancée, who was a young singer and former patient. The young couple thought that therapy for the young man's extremely high voice was now necessary since over the telephone he was invariably mistaken for a girl.

Examination of the larynx revealed healthy, well developed proportions with rather long and wide vocal cords. The voice was that of complete falsetto function (head-register).

The patient's father had died when he was twelve years old, but even when alive he did not play an important role in the boy's life. The patient grew up with four sisters, and his friends were their girl friends. He disclosed that at school he preferred to associate with girls as he felt more at home with them than he did with boys. It was obvious that no adequate father image had existed to mold his behavior during the crucial years of adolescence. Neither at home nor at school did he associate with a mature male, and his play life was such as to deprive him even of the slant which boyish games and sports could have given him. This made successful identification extremely hard for him. Well into his late teens his mother was the pivotal influence in his life. With the help of his fiancée his interests changed and he tried to free himself from the overintense family life. However, after four years' engagement, his mother still could not reconcile herself to the idea of his marriage and was still trying to separate the young couple.

This was the situation when the patient came for help. The mechanical part of therapy was comparatively simple. When the larynx is in good condition, exercises lower the pitch rapidly. Under slight finger pressure on the "Adam's apple" the patient clears his tone on a low pitch. This is always possible because again this coordination in the patient's mind is not connected with communication. This low pitch is used on a low vowel (o or oo) which the patient then prolongs into a long "o." During this procedure the patient's attention is called to the palpable chest resonance, which is absent during the use of falsetto voice. He therefore acquires a palpable control mechanism. The pitch reached is lower than the one which will be used later. The noise produced in clearing the throat is changed into a clear tone. Monotonous exercises (best in reading aloud) are performed, with syllables kept equally low, long, and loud on this newly acquired pitch. This helps to give the patient a new pattern through auditive, motor, kinesthetic association. In this particular case, Mr. J. R. after one day was unable to repeat his former pattern.

So far the treatment is simple unless complications develop at home. Chapter II describes the psychodynamics of mutation. Mr. J. R. came home with a true, low baritone voice and was promptly ridiculed by his mother who called him "bull-frog." She recognized immediately that she had lost the battle. The complete change of voice indicated to her that the pendulum between mother and girl had stopped swinging.

Case 10.

Mr. R. N. A., a 22 year old engineering student, complained of hoarseness, pressure symptoms in his throat, vocal fatigue. He suspected wrong use of voice because treatment for laryngitis had not helped him.

The larynx revealed marked redness and slight swelling, mainly along the free edges of the cords. Closure of the glottis was somewhat incomplete.

The voice was extremely high, almost completely in the head register. There was frequent throat clearing.

The patient told readily about his home life without being urged. He was fairly well adjusted to girls, had many dates, had never been "in love." He spoke with irritation of his mother, who "pries too much and wants to know what I do and think." During first conversations the patient avoided any mention of his father. It was a difficult subject to introduce, but immediately after it was the patient's facial expression changed entirely and he expressed profound hatred for his father. He gave a vivid picture of the man who knows everything better and "bullied" wife and son. The son's problem was undisguised and unrelieved hatred of his father. Identification was made difficult by the male parent's obnoxiousness. He hated everything about his father—including his deep voice. He admitted that he shaped his habits and manners deliberately opposite to those of his father and that he never permitted himself to "bellow in a deep voice."

Voice training had to be followed by psychiatric treatment because a deeper rooted neurosis was present. The psychodynamics are easily recognizable through vocal dynamics—the voice remains high because a low voice would represent the father who is hated.

CHAPTER VI

Vocal Features of Neurosis

IF IT IS TRUE that from the process of degeneration, disability and disease one may learn the nature of the parts that constitute the healthy whole, the previous case histories should, by throwing light on the vocal mechanisms of neurosis, also permit checking the validity of analytical hypothecations. Perhaps the first important general observation one makes is that voice falls apart much sooner than speech does. This is logical as it is more directly connected with emotional processes and less subject to cortical control.

Since by definition it is the logical organization of control that is missing in neurosis, the vocal apparatus, which mirrors all psychodynamic processes, must show signs of this lack of control. We find that hyper- and hypofunction or both, spasticity, and incoordination are such signs in certain contexts. The voice which is governed by rigid neurotic substitutions does not adapt itself fully to real emotional situations.

Pressure problems are most common. These may affect respiration or tensor or closing muscles in the vocal mechanism proper, or in the resonator. Uncertain intonation, unsure pitch, disturbed tonal continuity are some of the audible results. Fatigue is a consequence, though in some cases it engulfs the speaker from the very outset. It affects the intensity and pitch of the tone and is accompanied by a vague sensation of irritation. Neurotic strain and fatigue are sometimes accompanied by hyperesthesias in some part of the resonator. Mucus and dryness may alternate, and swallowing may plague the neurotic to an almost compulsive degree.

It a normal vocal coordination does not bring the expected result, by-paths may unconsciously be sought. Some of these are quite evident in singing. A singer may tiptoe when he sings a high tone. He may raise his eyebrows, open his eyes wide, wrinkle his forehead. Or he may use the muscles in chest or abdomen in a manner that has no relation whatsoever to tonal intensity or quality. Such neurotic movements must be distinguished from poor habits acquired through faulty training, though wrong training often leads singers to secondary neuroses.

The position of the larynx in vertical direction is important in many neurotic syndromes. The larynx is "suspended" in a balanced way between two muscle groups, one of which connects it upward to the hyoid bone, the other downward to the sternum. Neurotic pressure may disturb the balance, and the hyperfunction (or hypofunction) of one or the other muscle groups modifies the voice. For example, forced chest function exerts downward pressure on the larynx, which takes a relatively low position toward the chest. The trachea, a collapsible organ, becomes compressed in the process, and creates an as yet incompletely explored sound effect. Falsetto is produced with a high position of the larynx and a stretched trachea.

Breathiness of the voice is caused by incomplete closure of the glottis. Air which is destined for sound formation, for creating vibrations in the vocal cords, escapes unused—the "wild air."

In Chapter I, in the discussion of creative hearing, the tenor with the "dumpling in his throat" was mentioned. (Tenors seem to be afflicted by it more often than others.) The base of the tongue comes too close to the posterior pharyngeal wall and the tone sounds pressed and "narrow." The interesting component in this phenomenon is the self-deceit of the singer. This coordination gives him an overwhelming feeling of his own sound production, especially of the high tones. He "hears" a powerful sound while the audience hears no such thing. Moreover, the listeners get a tickling sensation in their throats which gives them laryngeal fidgets.

The most important vocal dysfunction in neurotic conditions is the use of wrong range, sometimes accompanied by separation of registers. Under conditions of deep anxiety the normal range is spurned and one that is symbolically more promising is favored. The process is called "introjection" in psychology. If one feels inferior, then behaving as if he is the "superior" individual with whom he desires to identify himself gives moral support. Hence the borrowed vocal range.

In adolescence, when insecurity and incomplete identification are physiologically conditioned, vocal insecurity and imitation are not neurotic. They become neurotic only if they persist to an age at which the individual should have succeeded in finding his own expression without resorting to introjection.

In vocal neurosis, professional neuroses might further be distinguished as a subcategory. They vary in nature. They may be caused by conflicts inherent in the profession and may leave vocal scars without being directly connected with voice production. Of course we are speaking here of professions in which the voice is a major tool and asset. The neurosis may in some cases stem directly from the function of phonation or be closely connected with it. One should not forget, however, that these professions which often severely tax the vocal apparatus may be subject to non-neurotic functional disorders, and these should not be confused with neurotic conditions.

ANXIETY

Fear and anxiety are perfectly normal reactions of the human organism. They become neurotic only when they govern the behavior pattern of the individual in inappropriate situations or if they defy control. There is scarcely any neurotic syndrome in which anxiety does not play a part. It attends also a good many psychoses as well as non-mental diseases.

All the symptoms of neurotic anxiety involve the vocal mechanism. To mention some: the "lump in the throat" feeling, uncontrollable weeping, air hunger, tension, fatigue. Audible symptoms run the gamut from a rough or wavering tone, through inspiratory phonation, to aphonia or mutism.

Respiratory processes are especially sensitive to fear and anxiety. Fear "settles" in the diaphragm and the coordination between diaphragmatic pressure and laryngeal pressure gets out of gear. Normally this coordination sustains the tone, but when respiratory pressure is weaker than pressure of the glottis (which holds the vocal cords together), the tone becomes a quavering tremolo. When the respiratory pressure is stronger than the pressure of the glottis, air escapes with an explosion, in glottal stroke, or it escapes as "wild air," which is not a real surplus since it should have been used for phonation.

Normally phonation is entirely on expiration. It is easy to check on what happens in inspiratory speech. All one has to do is to try it. The harder one tries, the worse the sound becomes. And if one presses hard enough, total aphonia results. There are other types of inspiratory voice. Some people interpolate tiny inspiratory movements while exhaling and speaking, and this makes the tone intensity flicker. A further variant is when the respiratory apparatus is kept in inspiratory position while the individual exhales and phonates. In singing this is achieved, after much training and practice, to obtain appoggio, tone support. When coordination is involuntary, the pressure is too weak to support the tone and tonal continuity is disturbed. Thus, considering only the element of breathing, the voice of anxiety will range from the breathy hoarseness of fear and annoyance to the inspiratory whisper of chronic worry. In between, as a kind of transition, is pseudo-appoggio.

However, it is not only the breathing mechanism which reacts to anxiety. Vocal cords are voluntary muscles which are subject to fear reactions. They are elastic; they can become shorter or longer; they can cramp and relax. In normal phonation the vocal cords touch one another in a relaxed leisurely way.

Aimless forms of nervous motor activity are primitive reactions to stimuli. Primitive organisms will move all over (or will freeze into immobility) when touched. The urge to remove inner tension by movement governs the organism in an undifferentiated manner. Selective, efficient reactions appear only at more highly developed levels. Human emotions have a component of awareness in addition to the mass of sensations and glandular or motoric reactions common to lower forms. Panic and hysterical tantrums are archaic reactions to which human beings regress under extreme internal or external pressure. A less pronounced form of undifferentiated motor reaction is the fidget. Constant throat clearing, frequent unconscious ejaculations, or insertions of stereotypes such as "you know," "O.K.," "you see," etc. and meaningless embolophrasias *(e-e-e, a-a-a)* are forms of vocal fidgets.

Acute fear, extreme anxiety or depression may inhibit or paralyze all or some motor functions. This is as archaic a reaction as aimless panic. Aphonia and mutism are vocal expressions of such emotional states.

Depression, indecision, and a vague sensation of unreality are often associated with anxiety neurosis. We discussed the highly limited vocal pattern of depression in some detail. Higher and higher rise the defensive walls around the expressional sources of the individual until only a narrow channel of escape is left. The next step may be aphonia.

Indecision and a vague feeling of unreality will make the voice too soft or occasionally too loud. The last syllable may be raised, twisting statements into questions, or it may be lowered to a murmur, leaving the listener guessing. The mucous membranes may become too dry; or when excitement replaces fear, they may be too moist, and in either case they modify resonance. When the aggressive component comes into ascendancy, sudden bursts of dynamics can be heard; words may be started with hard attack; last syllables may be strongly accented; or too many words crammed into one irregular breath. Occasionally overcautious enunciation is heard, reminiscent of the gingerly walk of the inebriate who is not quite sure that the environment will cooperate.

The general irritability and shifting of moods and the mixture of shyness, frustration and resentment which characterize anxiety neurosis are more evident from the voice than from any other behavior expression. Symbolically speaking, every forward step is followed by two backward ones. The impulse to talk carries the germ of inhibition in it, and the conflict invariably results in fatigue, which molds the pattern: loud fading into soft; high pitch sinking to low (maintaining the muscular effort needed for the high tone to too much effort); accents becoming indistinct toward the end; respiration more frequent; and so forth.

CONVERSION

Functional disturbances caused by mechanical abuse of the vocal cords may or may not be neurotic. Since however, the larynx is a secondary sex organ, it lends itself readily as a siding for neurotic conflicts of a sexual nature. Between these two poles of non-neurotic functional voice trouble and conversion in the strict psychoanalytic sense of the word, there is a wide gradation of possible organ neuroses. While these are as yet largely unexplored, certain significant facts have compelled attention. First, it seems that apparently negligible changes in external situations may produce, possibly through psychomotoric conditioning, violent disturbances in the organ functions of some people. Others seem unaffected by similar circumstances which they are capable of handling on a cerebral level. Looking from a different angle, it would seem as if the autonomic processes of some individuals are more susceptible to cerebral interference than are those of others. Hence the so-called disposition to peptic ulcer, spastic colitis, etc.

The respiratory system is especially sensitive to such cerebral inferences, complicated by the fact that, contrary to other autonomic processes, the respiratory and vocal muscles are voluntarily controlled.

The propensity for volitional control of the vocal apparatus is the secret of the "miraculous cures" in some voice disorders. It is possible to shock the patient into normal functioning by unexpected motor stimulation. For example, a laryngologist performs a routine tonsillectomy on a child. After three days the child has no pain but has typical open rhinolalia, speaking indistinctly, with a "stiff" soft palate. The mother, near hysteria, accuses the doctor of improper surgery and of ruining her child's life. The doctor eyes the little boy with disfavor or mild amusement, then makes him open his mouth, tells him to say *a-a-a,* and touches the inert soft palate with a cotton swab. The palate reacts promptly, the voice becomes normal. Everyone but the child is happy. Gone are ice cream, candy, pampering, stories; back to school and the everyday grind. If the child is not neurotic, his voice will remain normal. If he is neurotic, the "cure" will not take in the long run. Mechanical stimulation, suggestion, persuasion, hypnosis, all influence these voluntary muscular processes, but they do not affect the core of the neurotic disturbance.

Neuroses can occur in normal as well as in organically ill organs, or in organs that have been ill in the past. The term "disposition" is applied to organs which are apt to play host to neurotic symptoms which imitate or occasionally cause physical symptoms of some illness or disorder. The choice of organ is highly significant and in true conversion reveals much of the patient's deeper problems. But environmental influences, changing social trends, have much to do with the outward course of a neurosis and they often determine the choice of the organ "hosts."

With the growing influence of voice on our lives and the consequent increase in the professions and professionals whose tool in trade is voice, organ neurosis in the vocal mechanism is becoming more frequent.

Laryngeal organ neurosis, in addition to the previously noted peculiarities, differs from, let us say, spastic colitis in that it produces changes in function long before and to a greater degree than pain sensations. In this respect vocal neurosis resembles the neuroses of sense organs, such as the ear or the eye. The hysterical deaf person will not be racked by such pains as a middle-ear infection would inflict on him. And a neurotic aphonic does not necessarily "suffer" from hoarseness. This emphasis on functional modification rather than pain sensation has a deep psychological implication. Aphonia means "I don't want to express myself," just as hysterical deafness means, "I don't want to hear anything." However, in contrast to hysterical deafness or hysterical blindness, neurotic aphonia often reserves a small channel for expression. The patient is able to articulate in a voiceless whisper. Even in complete aphonia, gestures and writing may tell the story, and only in extreme cases does the "back door" to communication close completely.

Phylogenetically and ontogenetically voice production is autoerotic activity before it is communication. The infant derives pleasure from phonation as an oral activity, and secondarily he learns to derive pleasure from hearing himself. According to psychoanalytic theory those parts of infantile sexuality that are not integral to adult sexual life become transformed into character traits. Greediness, gluttony, restlessness, impatience, ambition are considered oral character traits. But much of the libidinous oral activity of early childhood is absorbed virtually unchanged into mature sexuality, and much is retained in original form in such pleasures as eating, speaking, singing. Little of it is sublimated. Yet in either form, sublimated or as an infantile libidinal vestige, oral libido may enter into neurotic complexes even to the degree of character neurosis. Overeating is an example of archaic orality; while on a more complex level, oral-sadistic tendencies of biting and swallowing (ingestion) may be transformed into vocal expressions of hostility and manipulativeness. Demanding, clinging individuals are fixated at an early infantile stage and extreme neurotic talkativeness may be the result of unsatisfied sucking needs.

The following case history shows how the already damaged larynx can play host to conversion:

Mrs. D. B., middle-aged, very impulsive and determined, had been treated three years previously for a non-malignant chest tumor by x-ray therapy. Seemingly the therapy and not the malignancy had injured the recurrent nerve, with resulting paralysis of the left vocal cord. She relearned to talk with an audible voice. However, after several weeks, she found her voice fading away more and more and ultimately she could talk only in a whisper. Her previous medical history was informative insofar as she had been operated upon six times before the advent of this latest chest disease and had had many lengthy sick periods of an indistinct nature.

Laryngoscopy showed the left vocal cord in cadaveric position whereas the right one moved freely. However, during closing function it did not reach the midline but stopped at about the same spot to which the left one had its fixation.

It is common experience that patients whose breathing apparatus becomes narrowed by pathology or surgery develop anxiety reactions. Though the narrowed passages are adequate for normal breathing, suffocating and choking sensations are felt until the patient gets used to his impairment. Intelligent explanation and reassurance usually help.

In Mrs. D. B.'s case the situation was more complicated. Here a floating anxiety induced by the paralysis of the left cord, and no doubt increased by the patient's generally neurotic tendencies, fastened itself to the intact right vocal cord. She did not have breathing difficulty but she did lose her means of vocal expression. One vocal cord was paralyzed for organic, the other for functional, reasons. The result was no communication except in a laborious whisper. Her stay on the West Coast was too short to get to the crux of her trouble. Treatments and training helped to reestablish function of the right vocal cord. The prognosis of sustained cure is none too hopeful, however.

It was mentioned earlier that aphonia can be the symbol of death. It may mean the wish to die or it may be a death wish directed against someone else. In other words, it is either a withdrawal or a self-punishment. The next case history shows how a student punished her singing teacher with her aphonia.

Miss R. L., aged 17 years, had been talking in a whisper, hardly audible, for over two years. No pathology was visible other than incomplete closure of the glottis.

Phonation was reestablished by a "clearing the throat" technique which after some days developed a well sustained tone from hard attack. It came out afterwards that J. was an exceptionally musical child, endowed with absolute pitch and with very excellent artistic taste. Two years before, she had started to disagree with her music teacher, whom she called lowbrow, in matters of taste. Besides, her own musical hearing was far superior since the teacher did not have absolute pitch. She felt that he kept her down compared with her own ambitious plans. Just about this time she caught a cold with some larynx involvement. She did not recover her voice. To begin with, it was a true adolescent protest. Then followed a wrong diagnosis (laryngitis), and the wrong psychological approach by her surroundings created a secondary anxiety neurosis which in a vicious circle prolonged the distressing symptoms. The symptoms disappeared after she became convinced that she still had an exceptional voice and that as an adult she could outgrow her immature revolt and could have the musical career of her own choosing.

It was her singer's personality, her oral libido, that chose the organ in which to create the symptom of protest.

The frustrated female voice is a widespread symptom in contemporary Western cultures, and because of the particular position which so many of its exponents hold it helps mold the voice of the younger generation. It contains a mixture of complaint and reproach. It is, first of all, a tense voice. Other acute emotions like fury and fear may create vocal tension. Frustration, however, is a long-lasting situation. Therefore, it imposes exaggerated muscular contraction which prevents easy phonation. The voice becomes higher, the resonator (the area between vocal cords and lips) is narrowed and the tone acquires a pressed quality. Besides the general hyperfunction of vocal muscles, auxiliary muscles are also drawn into helping phonation.

The seat of frustration, the process it affects most directly, is nasal resonance. Some ambivalence is found here. The lasting condition leads to shrinking of nasal mucous membranes, and the voice sounds cold, or more aptly, it lacks warmth. In acute situations, however, especially when self-pity and embarrassment come to the fore, the mucous membranes may swell and show symptoms of vasomotor disturbance, giving the effect of a complaining, tearful sound.

Because of the aggressive component inherent in frustration (reproach), melody is poor and range is limited. The intensity is rigid, due to the steadily forced hyperfunction. For the same reason there is little or no modulation of accents. One of the problems of neurotics is that they hear their own voices. Some become inebriated by the sound of their voices, some may be afraid of it. Their voices may symbolize conscience (approving or disapproving), which in psychotic extremes leads to projection in the form of hallucination. This psychological process lies at the base of the frustrated teacher's self-consciousness about the minus quality of her voice, for which she sometimes tries to compensate by a pseudo-pathos. Since by definition a neurotic will try to solve a situation by means that have failed in the past to solve similar situations, the frustrated woman will accentuate her vocal peculiarities in an attempt to bolster her ego and bridge the gap between herself and her pupils. Instead of the dignity inherent in true pathos, a frank expression of self-esteem and the relationship to others, her voice will be a mixture of noisy aggressiveness and the whining pseudo-pathos of being misunderstood and misused.

Individual variations on the theme may be contributed by the acid accents of the sadistic personality, by the oily and saccharine pseudo-sympathy of the overcompensated, and by the affectations of superiority, high culture, and so on, of the extremely insecure.

Since in many communities a teacher may not marry if she wants to hold her job, sexual frustration often accompanies professional frustration. This enhances certain factors in the vocal pattern but does not change it basically. The endocrine effect of sexual frustration on the voice is through its influence on nasal mucous membranes. Register, range, melody, rhythm will undergo changes due to psychological impact under frustration. Naturally, frustrated voices are more often heard in social groups that are governed by rigid taboos than in groups which allow varied emotional outlets.

Besides the typical puritanic voice there is the frustrated voice of the puritan's daughter expressing conflicts of right and wrong, taboo and guilt, with an audible aggressive component. Again it should be mentioned that the importance of these vocal problems is in its contagion, in its pattern-building. The child exposed to this influence in daily communication with a mother image is by no means pacified by the frustrated voice. He will be irritated, disturbed, frightened. But on the other hand, the teacher's pattern will become the child's pattern to express his own conflicts. It is by no means sexual frustration exclusively which is vocalized in such a typical way. It is the broader concept of frustration, including the "provider" even more than the matinee idol. The teen-age girl reveals these vocal symptoms when she has fewer dates than her girl friend, thereby not being able to compete with her, and not because she is not in love!

There is no doubt that the cure of the teacher's vocal neurosis is less the physician's than the community's problem. But it can be achieved only if the community changes its attitude; if the teacher is accepted socially, on her own merits as a human being. Only then will the task of teaching compensate for its shortcomings and disappointments.

SINGERS' NEUROSES

According to popular belief, singers are temperamental and prey to all kinds of nervous afflictions. While this is a gross exaggeration, it does not take too much imagination to conceive the many anxieties, fears and superstitions that do beset a performer who, rain or shine, must be in good voice when the curtain rises at 8:30. The singer creates his instrument every time he performs. He often envies the instrumentalist who, barring accidents, can depend on the condition of his piano or violin, who is not incapacitated by the slightest touch of cold or by sitting in a smoky room or by driving on a dusty road.

Yet few singers would change places with the instrumentalist. Music making is pleasure, but the most intense pleasure comes from making music with one's own body. Singing, furthermore, has the power to give erotic experience on the receiving as well as on the giving end. Creative hearing makes the audience identify itself with the singer. The singer gets pleasure from exercising his vocal cords and from hearing himself sing, and also from the audience's appreciation. In consequence, emotional upheavals play havoc with vocal art.

Neurotic disorders of the singing voice often start with respiratory problems, with spastic contractions of the diaphragm, reflex functions of fear, anger, shock, and through the vicious circle of breathing consciousness.

Excessive use of the voice may affect the thyroid gland by increasing the blood circulation through this tissue. Individuals vary in sensitivity, but in no case is this phenomenon pathological. Yet it gives the subjective sensation of a lump in the throat or choking, neither of which is encouraging to a singer even if he knows that it is nothing serious. Depression and elation are so closely correlated with thyroid activity that not too long ago such emotional states were ascribed directly to hyper- or hypothyroidism. Only lately did we come to understand that depression and elation can influence the functioning of the thyroid as much as the reverse.

Case History: Anticipation Neurosis

Miss D. G., aged 19 years, mezzo-soprano, very depressed, came to the office with her agitated mother. The young artist had caught a cold three weeks before, and had had voice trouble since. She felt tired and cried at the slightest provocation.

Examination of throat, larynx and nose gave normal results. The basal metabolism was minus 18.

In spite of her youth the girl had already made many successful public appearances. She was under the guidance of an understanding singing teacher. Since different conductors had already auditioned the patient, who could really look forward to a fine career, she was regarded among artists as being surrounded by a certain aura of expectation. A few weeks before the consultation, Miss G. had sung in a concert during her menstrual period. In addition she had been handicapped by a slight cold. She felt that her high notes were less than adequate and was more perturbed than the actual event warranted. Since then she had had increasing difficulty with her high tones, felt generally unwell and listless. It must be said that the patient lived under an increasing fear as to whether she could fulfill all the expectations built around her. From this occasional disappointment of not being in best voice, defeat with its cumulative effect started to produce an anxiety neurosis.

Here simple reassurance was insufficient. The patient had to go through a positive experience before the success of therapy could be expected. Reassurance with regard to the healthy condition of the vocal organs helps. The ancient singer's questions, "Are my cords white? Do they close?" had to be answered first. Then, in the doctor's office, the questionable range was sung. Every possible strain was avoided. After the so-called difficult tones could be performed satisfactorily several times, the authority of the physician was expressed in a proper way. He explained that not only the visible appearance but the audible function of the vocal cords was normal.

In case of neurotic vocal difficulties the laryngologist should never discharge the patient without having heard his voice. The smallest portable house organ is sufficient to indicate range and pitch. These cases of anticipation neurosis require patience and interest on the part of the therapist, and as soon as the singer is once victorious this new experience will overlap the accumulated fear of defeat.

The third common "starter" of singers' difficulties, in addition to respiration and thyroid, is the reactivity of the mucous membranes of the nose. Stage fright actually produces physical symptoms in the nose and throat, so that a singer is not unreasonable when he asks for medical help just a few minutes before the performance. Reassurance is the best medicine. This may come from the presence of the doctor, magic symbol of omnipotence, or it may come from the warming-up process, which is so aptly termed in slang, "getting in the groove." In either case, with reassurance, the mucous membranes of the nose become moist and vibrant again and restore the brilliance of the tones. Some singers get over stage fright as soon as the curtain is up while others need the entire first act to reach the peak of their performance. The former are the fortunate ones who have a close rapport with the audience and who draw strength from its presence. The others are more introverted and less receptive.

Neurotic tension in the throat muscles is a serious handicap to public speakers and actors as well as to singers. But the speaker who feels stone-dry may reach for a glass of water before he speaks more than a few words; or he may tell a funny story to get relaxed and to establish a link with the audience while incidentally clearing his mind of the interfering thoughts that helped create the tension. The actor cannot reach for water but he can concentrate on the words he says, on the meaning of the part, on the feelings he is supposed to impersonate. The singer has no recourse to any of these devices. All he has to give is the tone, and to be able to sing he must have relaxed throat muscles. To sing well he must be at ease, he must feel the keen edge of vitality and the pleasure of perfect control.

And this brings us to some of the deeper roots of singers' neuroses. The oral-narcissistic character of the singer makes it logical that neurotic conflicts, and certainly those rooted in traumas of early infancy, should use the larynx as a cathexis for the sex organs. Too little is known, however, in this regard to establish any theories at the present time for the simple reason that not enough analytical material on singers exists.

The laryngologist-patient situation is especially difficult with singers. Semantically they do not understand each other. Body sensations in singing as explained by the singer appear to be entirely illogical to the physician. They are often mistaken for illusions, for sense perception with subjective perversion of objective content. In reality the sensation is illogical only because the self-localization is impossible—resonance is felt in sinuses, over special parts of the back, as anyone can find out for himself by singing.

The artistic temperament must be considered. The larynx is the most important organ for the singer, singing the most important function, and every performance is THE most important one of his whole career. Here the narcissistic attitude is not a deviation of personality, but it is often the thing which makes the singer. Laryngologists frequently have a negativistic attitude towards singers. They are often even hostile, paternalizing. This is because they did not learn to analyze a voice during their own training, they do not go often enough to singing recitals, and they have only an average knowledge of singing, which frequently means none. Too many times the physicians mention to singers an unimportant deviation of the septum or tonsil tags or plugs as the cause of acute vocal difficulty. The pontifical attitude expressed in the counsel, "You cannot sing; you need voice rest" completes the damage. How can one tell whether a singer suffering from anxieties expressed in vocal fatigue will actually benefit from resting his voice? Just the opposite may well occur. Vocal inactivity is frustration in itself. Expectation of what the result will be is usually followed by an even greater vocal breakdown.

In order to treat these so-called nervous disturbances in singers, the laryngologist should familiarize himself not only with the basic principles of singing, but he can actually benefit from taking lessons himself before he discusses the problems of singing with professionals. He should know the repertoire of the individual artist. How else can he know whether a singer is able to sing his part or not?

Only then, along with a reassuring attitude, can the physician become a guide for the singer. The singer will feel that he is in the hands of a therapist who understands his personal needs. The laryngologist to whom voice means the same for mailman and singer alike will not meet the singer's needs. From the therapeutic viewpoint it has to be stressed that certain medications are dangerous for singers. Cocaine, codeine, adrenaline cause dryness and stiffness of vocal cords. Silver nitrate should never be used on the singer's pharynx or larynx.

The singer's fear of tonsillectomy is mainly the result of bad experiences with colleagues. The greatest handicap to maintaining ideal vocal conditions is the possibility of scar result on the soft palate. This occasionally causes initial rigidity and stiffness. The best way of avoiding this rigidity is to start the following exercise two weeks after tonsillectomy.

Repeat often in staccato rhythm: nga, nge, ngee, ngoo, ngo. This will restore the flexibility of the soft palate in a short time. If the flexibility is missing, the singer will suffer from great anxiety concerning his future because of the change in resonance. The sound will be nasal, registers will be hard to blend.

COMPULSION-OBSESSION

Psychoanalytic theory holds that compulsion, both in the acute and chronic form, is an illness of persons who, through experiences in that stage of infantile development when excretory functions are of focal interest, have acquired a predisposition to anal-sadistic regression (Karl Abraham). (In simple words, their toilet-training was not constructive.) In contrast to infantile oral eroticism, a large part of infantile anal eroticism undergoes transformation into character traits and becomes sublimated. The original cathexes are replaced by a variety of symbols. Yet the basic reactions connected with retention and gradual or explosive relief remain the same (Fenichel).

Persistence, orderliness, secretiveness, aloofness, reserve and also procrastination are judged to be anal character traits; *i.e.,* they are supposedly developed as reaction formations to, or sublimations of, infantile anal eroticism. In pathological development, anal traits are often mixed with oral traits, since regression does not stop on a dot. Neither do developmental periods begin and end abruptly; they overlap for considerable periods.

As with other patterns of behavior, the compulsive individual will have a set vocal pattern. If he has vocal mannerisms, and he probably will have them, these will be heard regularly in response to certain stimuli. He may pause significantly between sentences. He surveys his thoughts as he does his possessions, to make sure they are displayed in the intended order. Some people not only arrange their thoughts but their sound production as well. If the tongue does not touch the exact spot it should when making a certain sound, they will repeat the movement until the exact spot is reached. The result is not merely a pause, but it is a pause full of preliminary movement, like crouching and tensing before jumping or winding up before pitching. The word does not come out before expiration and the vocal cord closure is carefully arranged, producing a pedantic, precise way of speaking.

Coprolalia is a term applied to the compulsive use of taboo words. Extreme guilt feelings at the intended or actual use of such words indicate the reverse side of the same coin. A great many of the taboo words in every language refer to basic body functions and often resemble body sounds emitted in connection with these functions. This onomatopoeia is of help in training infants who at first are encouraged to produce such body noises which are imitated to establish the association. Later, the functions are disciplined, as are the noises, and the infantile words and sounds first used for encouragement are now used for restraint in training. To the first simple associations of release and pleasure are now added displeasure, guilt, resentment and rebellion, as well as a desire to retaliate for the inflicted discomfort. However, this basic vocabulary of body functions is the foundation for the future use of what we term "four-letter words."

In the compulsion neurotic's subconscious, words may take the place of deeds and coprolalia in either positive or negative form is a frequent reduction of general or particular hostility. However, from our point of view a more interesting phenomenon occurs when the neurotic succeeds in controlling his words. He may even control the general intensity of his voice, which in our culture is consciously associated with expression of anger and hostility. Yet, since voice is primary to speech, some aspects of it escape cortical control, and the particular type of compulsion betrays itself in the character of certain sounds basic to onomatopoeic taboo words. Resentment may hiss in the *s* or spit in the hard attack of *f* and *p*.

Many compulsion neurotics use embolophrasias reminiscent of infantile vowel stuttering to fill up pauses between articulate speech. This type of sound insertion differs from the vocal substitutes for coprolalia. Though different in purpose and sound effect, it is akin to the winding up process for articulation. The neurotic signifies that he is not through speaking, that he continues to think and is now arranging his thoughts properly so as to present them with perfect precision. These embolophrasias are comparable to the small motions with which a compulsive pushes his watch and pencil hither and thither on the night table until they are in the very spot and at the correct angle he intended.

Giggling is another vocal compulsion. The fact that preadolescent girls are addicted to it (and at that stage it should not be considered neurotic) suggests that in adults it might indicate a regression to the urethral rather than to the anal-erotic stage of presexual development. Giggling has a marked component of "letting flow," combined with a high watery pitch. The increased existence of overtones causes this audibly liquid character. It is an almost exclusively female expression and when observed in men, a symptom of femininity.

VOCAL CORD NEUROSIS

In contrast to vocal neurosis, in the neurosis of the vocal cord itself we find conversion symptoms which are visually recognizable in true pathological tissue changes. The vocal changes are of a secondary nature.

Contact ulcers of vocal cords are observed frequently. It is textbook opinion that they are almost always caused by faulty use of voice. This may be right for a certain percentage, but it is a very small one. Even were the voice recognized as too high or too low, the psychodynamics still would have to be explained. And then it would become evident that even in these cases which are attributed to the wrong use of voice, a neurotic component would be involved.[54, 55] The same would be valid in an allergic origin which again would have a psychosomatic stamp, especially when the larynx is the only seat of allergic manifestation. In considering neurotic origin the most important factor is the large number of contact ulcer patients with previously normal voices. The following example is most illustrative.

A singer who developed a large contact ulcer on the typical location (posterior end of the left vocal cord) was examined the day before a concert. Twenty-four hours previously he had watched his car roll down a hill and hit another car, with little damage. But this anxiety on a day which was already emotionally overloaded must have caused the ulcer, because it disappeared completely within forty-eight hours.

Since the skin rash of a baby is considered a protest expressed in *body* language, we need to understand more thoroughly allergic manifestations in the larynx, the *organ of expression* itself.

A boy, aged 9, son of an ice cream manufacturer, had been almost aphonic for three years. He spoke only in a high, pressed whisper. His vocal cords were slightly edematous and revealed symmetrical nodes between anterior and middle third of the cords. He was allowed to indulge in all his father's merchandise, including candy bars, and had certainly made the most of this opportunity. Elimination diet and anti-histamine helped to some extent in shrinking the nodes and the edema. The voice, however, and the visible pathology were cured only after the patient had expressd his resentment, amounting almost to hatred, against his older brother. Fortunately this conflict could be eliminated. It completed the cure.

Conclusion

THIS BOOK HAS DEALT WITH vocal analysis and its use for the interpretation of the normal and neurotic personality. The more serious disorders of personality have been mentioned only in passing. Some preliminary comments on the voice of psychosis can be made here. The author is currently making a thorough investigation into this aspect of voice and the results will ultimately be published.

There are marked differences between neurotic and psychotic vocal expression. When one finds neurotic vocal symptoms in a psychotic patient, this usually means that neurosis is mixed with the psychosis. The neurotic symptom of stuttering in a schizophrenic signifies that both conditions can coexist. In *schizophrenics* we find the following vocal symptoms:

(1) Rhythm is prevalent over melody. A rhythmic repetition of vocal patterns is characteristic.

(2) Registers are often separated: isolated head-register is used for long periods, often for days. The use of mixed registers probably accompanies temporarily successful communication.

(3) Complete absence of melisms. This represents the inability of the patient to express appeal.

(4) Decreased nasal resonance.

(5) Melody is never "gliding" but always jumping in intervals, often without any correlation to content.

(6) Mannerisms are used in histrionic excess. When such a patient uses the voice of authority, it is almost a burlesque of the voice of authority.

(7) Accents are inappropriate to the content of his speech. This is part of a constantly repeated rhythmic pattern which is maintained in an almost compulsive way (this symptom can never be found in *neurotic voices*).

In summary, the basic characteristics of schizophrenic expression is the use of rhythmic patterns, verbal as well as vocal ones. Words which are seemingly meaningless are interpolated regularly, other words are used over and over again. The patient seems gripped by rhythmical patterns of vocal intensities which he cannot escape. Even the divergence of registers occurs in a certain rhythmic pattern, now head-register, then chest or mixed registers. The use of isolated head register gives to the male voice a marked feminine character, whereas the chest register emphasizes the male quality of the voice. It is as if the patient wishes to achieve fusion of the two sexes—it has been suggested* that the schizophrenic attempts to achieve the hermaphrodite ideal, and it is interesting how clearly this appears in his voice.

The remarkable splitting of registers by schizophrenics the author prefers to call *schizophonia*.

Ventriloquism

Since the schizophrenic seems to speak in two voices, schizophrenia brings to mind ventriloquism where "the other personality" is externalized almost in the flesh and sits on the obsessed's arm or lap to contradict him, fight him, warn him; in short, to do everything that voices tell the schizophrenic. In former centuries divine oracles were proclaimed through ventriloquism and until the beginning of modern times a supernatural origin was believed.

The physiology of ventriloquism consists of use of higher range.[56, 57] Expiration is minimized. Articulation occurs with lips closed as much as possible. The trick consists in lowering of the epiglottis, and in narrowing of the resonator (the space between lips and vocal cords). Resonatory proportions undergo a change through these coordinations so that the voice seems to come from farther away. The softer stream of expiratory air causes only partial vibrations of vocal cords, thus using only higher overtones.

The personality of the ventriloquist is the center of interest. It is not so much "How to Learn Ventriloquism?" as "Who Learns It?" There is little doubt that the love and hatred between speaker and dummy has become one of the most evident manifestations of schizoid expression.

In contrast to the schizophrenic voice, the voice of the manic-depressive patient reveals as the predominant factor complete absence of exaggerated rhythmic patterns. Instead the speech melody gains increased importance. In depressive periods the range shrinks, and is increased in manic phases. The nasal resonance is marked, giving to the voice a "warmer" feeling. The melody glides through the pitches, the intervals are hardly ever jumpy. Accents often have a more musical nature, while the dynamic character of the accent decreases.

The depressed voice is often described as monotonous, but under exact analysis it can be seen that the typical feature is not the monotony, but the uniformity, the regular repetition of the same gliding down interval. When the tone goes down, the intensity decreases proportionately. In the schizophrenic voice the intensity never decreases with the lowering pitch. Manic conditions express themselves vocally through uncontrolled intensities, extremely wide range which "stretches" registers, and highly dynamic accents often accompanied by fast tempo of speech. There is no appeal through pathos or melisms, and no esthetic balance of the whole mosaic of acoustic dimensions.

To conclude these brief remarks on the voice of psychosis, we must emphasize that although the vocal features are different in psychosis and neurosis, the same analytical technique can be applied.

VOICE THERAPY

Voice problems which are caused by inflammatory conditions of the larynx certainly require treatment by medication. Functional disturbances, *e.g.*, recurrent paralysis of the vocal cord, will be helped by physiotherapy, by exercises, vibration massage, use of Faradic current. If laryngeal allergy influences phonation, anti-allergic treatment is indicated; however, in all of these conditions, the emotional factors might be the precipitating cause and the laryngologist must be aware of this. However, the patient comes to the laryngologist and voice specialist because he has a complaint about his vocal apparatus. He does not see the laryngologist to get rid of a phobia, a compulsion, an anxiety or other neurosis. Were the same patient to seek psychiatric advice primarily, he would disclose his nervous symptoms together with whatever physical symptoms were bothering him. But even when the patient comes unwillingly and under pressure from his family, his very protest will be focused on the overt symptom. For instance, take the problem of neurotic aphonia. The therapist can be annoyed or stern. Through the impact of fear, he may frighten the patient into speaking again. Or he may employ gentler methods. But whether the patient continues to use his newly found voice or relapses into voiceless whispering, the problem remains: What made him lose his voice in the first place?

The person who was frightened into speaking again by a stern, down-to-earth practitioner may continue to speak, and develop instead another spastic symptom, such as diarrhea, which will enable him to take his symptoms to a more sympathetic physician; or he may be obstinate and lapse again into whispering, thus thumbing his nose at the victorious laryngologist. There is no guarantee that gentler methods are more effective in the long run. Treatment really should start where it usually ends—when the patient regains his voice.

Most laryngologists are afraid to trespass in a field not their own. Yet if he wants solid results in the treatment of functional disorders, many of which are of a neurotic character, the laryngologist must treat his patient as a whole and not merely as the possessor of a single organ or organ group. He must couple whatever physical treatments are in order with a psychotherapeutic approach. To help a patient whose vocal troubles are neurotic in origin, the laryngologist must acquire the knowledge that will enable him to do this in a professional manner and not as a dilletante. It is less important that he formally classify the neurosis than that he do the same thing as the psychotherapist—find the underlying emotional conflicts and help the patient become aware of their effect on his voice.

Bibliography

1. Jones, Harold E.: Development in Adolescence. New York, D. Appleton-Century Co., 1943. 122-123.
2. Moses, Paul J.: The study of voice records; Jones, Harold E.: The analysis of voice records. Journal of Consulting Psychology. 6:255-261, 1942.
3. Lloyd, Wilma, et al.: Analysis and Interpretation of the Creative Work of John Sanders. Confidential Publication, Inst. of Child Welfare, University of California Study of Adolescence, 1942.
4. Froeschels, E.: Psychogenic impediments of the voice. Laryngoscope 49:1225-1230, 1939.
5. Biehle, Herbert: Die Stimmkunst. Leipzig, Kistner & Siegel, 1931.
6. Pear, T. H.: Voice and Personality. London. Chapman & Hall, 1931.
7. Bühler, Karl, in H. Herzog: Stimme und Persönlichkeit. Ztschr.f.Psychol. 130:300-309, 409-413, 1933.
8. Cantril, H., and Allport, G. W.: The Psychology of Radio. New York, Harper and Brothers, 1935.
9. Sanford, Fillmore: Voice and personality. Psychological Bulletin 39: 837, 1942.
10. Scripture, E. W.:Anwendung der Graph.Methode auf Sprache u.Gesang. Leipzig, J. A. Barth, 1927.
11. Weiss, Deso: Ganzheitsforschung u.exper.Phonetik. Mitteil.über Sprach-u. Stimmheilk. Vol. II. 9-10, Vienna, D. Weiss, 1936.
12. Bernfeld, Siegfried: Über Faszination, Imago, XIV. 1928.
13. Paget, R.A.S.: Human Speech. London, Kegan Paul, 1930. p. 132; This English. London, Kegan Paul, 1935. pp. 26-34.
14. Bühler, Karl: Sprachtheorie. Jena, G. Fischer, 1934.
15. Moses, Paul J.: Vocal analysis. Arch. Otolaryngol. 48:171-186, 1948.
16. Wolff, Werner: The Expression of Personality. Experim. Depth Psych. New York, Harper, 1943. (Chapt. III: Voice and Personality).
17. Wolff, Werner: The Threshold of the Abnormal. New York, Hermitage House, 1950.
18. Flatau, Theod. S., and H. Gutzmann: Die Stimme des Säuglings. Arch. f.Lar. u.Rhin.Berlin, Hirschwald. 18:139-151, 1906.
19. Froeschels, E.: Pathology and therapy of stuttering. In Twentieth Century Speech and Voice Correction. New York, Philosophical Library, 1948.
20. Stinchfield Hawk, Sara: Speech Therapy of the Physically Handicapped. Stanford, Stanford University Press, 1950. pp. 128-129.
21. Weiss, Deso: The pubertal change of the human voice. Fol. Phoniatrica. II. 3: 132, 1950.
22. Nadoleczny, Max: Lehrbuch der Sprach-und Stimmheilkunde. Leipzig, F. C. W. Vogel, 1926. p. 195.
23. Moses, Paul J.: Social adjustment and voice. Quart. J. Speech. 27: 532-536, 1941.

24. Faulkner, William B.: The effect of emotions upon diaphragmatic function. Psychosomatic Med. Vol. 3:2, 1941.

25. Schilling, R.: Inner speech and speech development. Bericht deutsch.Ges. f.Sprachheilk. 94-98. Berlin, J. Springer.

26. Draper, George, C. W. Dupertuis, J. L. Caughey: Human Constitution in Clinical Medicine. New York, Paul B. Hoeber, 1944. pp. 75-93.

27. Abraham, Karl: Contributions to the Theory of the Anal Character. Selected Papers. London, Inst. of Psychoanalysis and Hogarth Press, 1927.

28. Abraham, Karl: Psychoanalytische Studien zur Characterbildung. Leipzig, Internat.Psychoanalytischer Verlay, 1925.

29. Sievers, Eduard: Grundzüge der Phonetik. Leipzig, Breitkopf u.Härtel, 1901.

30. Bernstein, F.: Stimme u.Erblichkeit. Proceedings of the Internat. Congress of Phonetic Sciences. Amsterdam, 1932.

31. Iro, Otto: Diagnostik der Stimme. Wien, Verlag Die Stimmbildung, 1923.

32. Kretschmer, Ernst: Physique and Character. New York, Harcourt, Brace, 1936.

33. Sheldon, W. H.: The Varieties of Human Physique. New York, Harper and Brothers, 1940.

34. Moses, Paul J.: Konstitution u.Stimme in ihrer charakterologischen Beziehung Zitschr.Hals,Nas.Ohrenheilk. 30:1, 1931.

35. Moses, Paul J.: Experimental-phonetische Grundlagen einer Charakterologie der Stimme. Transactions First Meeting Internat. Society f.Experimental Phonetics.Bonn,1930.

36. Holmes, Thomas H., Helen Goodell, Stewart Wolf, Harold Wolff: The Nose. Springfield. Charles C Thomas, 1950.

37. Koblanck, Alfred: Die Nase als Reflexorgan. Vienna, Urban & Schwarzenberg, 1930.

38. Gajard, Dom Joseph: The Rhythm of Plainsong According to the Solesmes School. New York. J. Fischer & Brothers, 1943.

39. Fliess, W.: Die Nasale Reflexneurose. Wiesbaden, Bergmann, 1893.

40. Kafka, I.: Handbuch der vergleichenden Psychologie. Munich, Reinhardt, 1922. p. 206.

41. Pavlov, Michel: Origin of the sense of rhythm. de psychol. norm. et pathol. 8:719, 1924.

42. Helmholtz, Herm. Die Lehre von den Tonempfindungen. Braunschweig, Vieweg, 1913.

43. Faust, F.: Speech disorders and personality development. Allgem.Ztschr.f.Psychiatrie. 115:105, 40.

44. Stockert, F. G.: Über den Umbau und Abbau der Sprache bei Geistesstörung. Berlin, Karger, 1929. p. 9.

45. Schoen, Max: Psychology of Music. New York, Ronald Press, 1940.

46. Klages, Ludwig. Handschrift und Charakter. Leipzig, J. A. Barth. 1923.

47. Saudek, Robert: The Psychology of Handwriting. New York, G. Doran, 1926.

48. Grimme, H.: Sprachmelodik und Syntax. Proceedings First Meeting of Internat.Society f.Experim.Phonetics.Bonn,1930.

49. Fenichel, Otto: The Psychoanalytical Theory of Neurosis. New York, W. W. Norton & Co., 1945.

50. Ruesch, Jurgen and Gregory Bateson: Communication. The Social Matrix of Psychiatry. New York, W. W. Norton, 1951. p. 88.

51. Menninger, Karl A.: The Human Mind. New York. Knopf., 1946.

52. Dalma, G.: Körperbau and Psychose. Ztschr.f.d.ges.Neur.u. Psychiatrie. 97: 5, 1925.

53. Porta, Giovanbattista: De Humana Physiognomia, Libri IV. Rouen, 1650. (German Translation, Stuttgart, Hippocrates Verl. 1930).

54. Moses, Paul J.: Speech and voice therapy in otolaryngology. Eye, Ear, Nose & Throat Monthly 32:367-375, 1953.

55. Moses, Paul J.: The Psychosomatic Aspect of Vocal Analysis. Proceedings First Institute on Voice Pathology. Cleveland Hearing and Speech Center, Western Reserve University, 1952.

56. Luchsinger, R.: Über die Bauchrednerstimme. Folia Phoniatrica. 1:117-123, 1948.

57. Reich, W.: Ventriloquism. Ciba Journal, October 1950.

Index